JOURNEY *of* *the* HEART

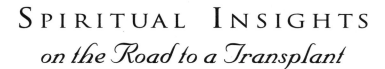

SPIRITUAL INSIGHTS
on the Road to a Transplant

JOURNEY of
the HEART

—❧—

SPIRITUAL INSIGHTS
on the Road to a Transplant

ELIZABETH ANN BARTLETT

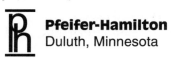

Pfeifer-Hamilton
Duluth, Minnesota

Pfeifer-Hamilton Publishers
210 West Michigan
Duluth, MN 55802-1908

218-727-0500
http://www.wholeperson.com/~books
E-mail: phbooks@wholeperson.com

Journey of the Heart: Spiritual Insights on the Road to a Transplant

7/97

Printed in the United States of America

10 9 8 7 6 5 4 3 2 1

Editorial Director: Susan Gustafson
Manuscript Editor: Kathy DeArmond-Lundblad

Library of Congress Cataloging-in-Publication Data

Bartlett, Beth, 1952–
    Journey of the heart : spiritual insights on the road to a transplant.
    192 p. 23 cm.
     ISBN 1-57025-128-2
     1. Bartlett, Beth, 1952—Health. 2. Heart—Transplantation—Patients—United States—Biography. I. Title.
RD598.B377 1996
362.1 '97420592'092—dc20   96-10148
{B}   CIP

V

For my heartmates

David and Paul

and

J.

Contents

In appreciation

I would like gratefully to acknowledge the many who helped me in the writing of this book. First and foremost, this book was in many ways the inspiration of my minister, Kathy Nelson, who first invited me to speak on the spiritual dimensions of my transplant experience. She, in a sense, called this book into being. My thanks as well to those who listened to me speak and encouraged me to put my thoughts into a book. Kathy also read initial drafts of some of the chapters and continued to be encouraging throughout the process.

My thanks also to my sister, Jeannie, and my brother Bruce for their love and support in this endeavor as they read initial drafts of some of the early chapters. Thanks as well to Sofia Ormaza for her guidance and counsel on the medical aspects of this book.

I am very grateful to the Dean of the College of Liberal Arts at the University of Minnesota-Duluth, Harry Hellenbrand, who graciously supported me in the writing of this book and who, along with his wife, Donna Hellenbrand, read, critiqued, and commented on the complete draft of the book. Their insights have made it a better book, and I thank them for that.

My thanks to Susan Gustafson at Pfeifer-Hamilton, who responded so enthusiastically to my initial proposal for the book that I felt heartened to go ahead and write it, and who has subsequently given her editing skills, thoughtfulness, and sensitivity to its completion. My thanks as well to all of those at Pfeifer-Hamilton who have helped to bring this book into being. My sincere gratitude to Don and Nancy Tubesing, who have been so enthusiastic and unwavering in their support of this project.

And to my husband, David, who believed in me and celebrated with me, and my son, Paul, who inspired so much of this book, my gratitude for their love and presence in my life.

Finally, to the many, many who did so much to keep me alive in body and spirit so that I could write this book, my heartfelt gratitude, especially to my donor, J., and her family, who more than anyone, have made this book possible. May this be a gift to you as well.

Journey of the heart

The story I am about to share is really two stories.

The first story tells of the sudden and severe worsening of a heart condition that had plagued me all of my adult life. It is the story of struggle with life-threatening illness, a struggle that was to culminate in a heart transplant.

The second is a story that we all share—a story of our common journey through the fears, doubts, and despair, as well as the joys, hopes, and wonder of life. It is a story told around my personal experience of illness, death, and new life, but it is more the story of our common human condition than of my individual heart condition.

This book began with a request from my minister to give a talk about the spiritual insights I had gained from my transplant experience. She and other people who have listened to my story encouraged me to gather these insights into a book. As I began writing the book, I brought together thoughts from my journals, reflections on my experience from a retrospective and introspective mirror, and wisdom from the songs and poetry and essays that have nurtured me throughout my life.

Though I wrote separate chapters on letting go and patience and hope and joy and gratitude and all the rest, as I continued, I found the distinctions among these qualities became blurred. Each one entails so much of all the others. Ultimately, they all seem to be speaking to the same truth.

The qualities elaborated on here are not the only or even the most important spiritual qualities. They are just the ones that presented themselves most clearly to me as I reflected on my experience. A doctor once jokingly remarked to me during a routine posttransplant biopsy that a heart transplant is the process of giving a new heart and then taking it away piece by piece. From a spiritual perspective, however, a transplant gives new insights—piece by piece.

In many ways, the insights gathered here are very old. Lessons of letting go, patience, humility, gratitude, hope, and joy recur throughout ancient spiritual traditions. What I bring to them is the lived experience of them and reflections on their meaning in the context of my life—a life about to end and a life about to begin. They are valuable lessons and deserve a retelling.

I do not claim any privileged spiritual wisdom. Indeed, as I wrote, I struggled with what appeared to be my own arrogance and hypocrisy in writing a book on spiritual wisdom. But I have had a rare opportunity in this life—to live life on the edge of death, to venture into death, and then to experience second birth; to be both very old and very young in the middle ages of my life. My situation has enabled me to gain a perspective on life unavailable to most people except at the beginning, when they are too young to articulate it, or at the end, when there is no more time to pass it on. It has brought me incredible gifts, crystals of wisdom and insight, which I am eager to give to others. In no sense are the insights presented here the whole of spiritual wisdom. They are part of a journey, a journey of the heart.

My story

On May 4, 1990, I kissed my husband and baby boy good-bye and left to join my friends Jody and Mary at the Women's Coffeehouse. We had been making music together for several years, and once again it was time for our spring concert.

They tell me I played my heart out . . .

I woke up in a hospital bed with my husband, David, weeping at my side. My sister, Jeannie, was there too. I didn't understand. Why was I there? Why was Jeannie there? Where was my baby?

I apparently had suffered a cardiac arrest while performing at the coffeehouse. Fortunately, a doctor and two emergency-room nurses were in the audience. They gave me CPR and got me through the immediate crisis until paramedics came and took me to the hospital. The whole of the coffeehouse audience, along with other friends—including my dear neighbor, Nancy, who was on duty that night and walked in to find me in the coronary intensive care unit—kept vigil for days as doctors and nurses struggled to keep me alive.

I was not an easy patient. I fought so hard to get the ventilator tube out that it took six people to hold me and strap me down. My heart was as wild as my will and resisted almost all efforts to stabilize it. With persistence and prayers, I came around enough to be helicoptered to the Twin Cities, and there I awoke to find my life drastically changed.

This wasn't totally out of the blue. I had dealt with cardiac dysrhythmia all of my adult life. Nearly twenty years earlier, at the age of twenty, what I thought was a bad case of the flu turned out to be inflammations of the liver and the myocardium, the lining around the heart. I was hospitalized, became comatose, and came very close to dying. In the final hours, only my father's medical wisdom and persistence pulled me back from death's clutches. I recovered from that first acute bout with heart disease in three months' time, though I continued to have persistent heart dysrhythmia, which over the course of the next year slowly began to worsen. My doctor tried a lot of medications for the dysrhythmia, but nothing really helped, and about a year after my first brush with death, I collapsed in cardiac arrest. Revived, I was again hospitalized with life-threatening heart dysrhythmia. Again, I survived the crisis, but it was time to call in the specialists. I was sent to Ann Arbor, Michigan, where a doctor who specialized in cardiac dysrhythmia discovered what he called a "pseudoaneurysm"—a massive scarring on my left ventricle, the major pumping chamber of the heart—but no other deterioration of the heart or coronary arteries. He prescribed the appropriate medication, and soon my heart stabilized, and my life went on as usual. After several years, with a regular routine of exercise, I was able to wean myself off the medication entirely, and pronounced myself "cured."

My first inkling that something might still be amiss with my heart came fifteen years later in March of 1988. I was Jazzercising, which I had done regularly for about three years, when I felt my heart go into tachycardia (a rapid heart rate; there is a subtle yet clearly recognizable feel to it). The music and room began to fade, and then I fainted. I was out only briefly—my heart converted to a normal rhythm on its own—but I was scared. I was afraid to sleep that night and for several nights thereafter, but nothing more happened, and I eventually dismissed the episode as a fluke. Perhaps I had been overtired. Perhaps I had the flu.

Newly married, my husband, David, and I went ahead with our

plans to have a child. My pregnancy was fairly uncomplicated, except for some rough moments around the seventh month when I longed for a few steady heartbeats in a row. My doctor seemed to think little of it. My labor was long, but relatively uneventful. A string of potentially life-threatening premature ventricular contractions (PVCs) had doctors and nurses hovering and scurrying and pumping me with lidocaine, but I was oblivious to it all. My babe and I were in our own world, following our own rhythm—and then there he was. That cry was the sweetest sound I have ever heard.

We did it! We defied the odds and the doctors. They told me I couldn't, shouldn't, have children, but I knew that I could and I should. We did it! And here he was, my precious baby boy. I was born for this.

The next day my heart doctor talked to me about how I might be heading for a heart transplant. I wanted to shout, "Get out of here! This is my time to celebrate. Transplant! How absurd!" I denied it.

Two months later I was coughing up blood. The X rays showed my heart was bigger. My doctor thought I might have a year.

David's mother died that day.

A few weeks later, my visit to the transplant doctor at the University of Minnesota Hospital brought me hope. He said that although on paper I looked bad, in person I looked fine, and as long as I was feeling good and not experiencing any symptoms, I needed no treatment.

I returned home, focused on my baby and on healing my heart. I began to see a holistic healer. I meditated and visualized. I began to feel stronger and more confident. My blood pressure went way down. I was teaching, hiking, and feeling strong. We celebrated our baby's first birthday . . . and then came the coffeehouse concert.

So, waking up in a hospital bed on that day in May 1990 didn't take me by complete surprise. Indeed, I took it in stride. More than that, I was defiant. As far as I was concerned, I was fine. I'd lived with this all of my life. Being in the hospital was a nuisance. I just wanted to go home to my baby; my doctors thought otherwise.

To assess the irritability of my heart and the ability of various drugs to stabilize its rhythm, doctors at the University Hospital performed an electrophysiology study. It showed that drugs would be of little help in controlling my heart rhythm. I was quite opposed to drugs at the time in any event, and the only one that seemed to offer any hope—amiodarone—could also cause lung problems and congestive heart failure. I laughed at the very thought of taking that medication.

I did, however, accept having an automatic implantable defibrillator cardioverter implanted in my body. The device would monitor my heart rhythm and deliver an electric shock to convert a dangerous ventricular tachycardia to a normal sinus rhythm. This seemed a fairly innocuous solution. They said that the shock wouldn't hurt much, and I was certain that I would never need the shock. At least it wouldn't poison me . . . I was not prepared for the enormous implications of my decision.

My recovery from the surgery was very difficult. I had never known such pain, and every medication to relieve the pain made me sick. I was wounded in spirit as well as in body. Before the operation, I had felt strong and confident. Afterwards, I was weak, debilitated, scared. My body had never suffered such devastation. I'd been cut open and pried apart. I had wires all through me, and the Walkman-sized defibrillator stuck out in a huge lump just under my ribs. I hated it.

And it seemed to hate me. We were at war, and we fought for four years. They say it saved my life, but I'm not at all convinced.

The first time it shocked me I had been home from the hospital for only one day. I was so weak. Just the little bit extra I was called to do in climbing the stairs into my house and being up and about caused me such pain I couldn't eat or sleep. Simply walking from one room to another made my heart race. Late that first night, as I turned the corner into my room, I felt my heart rate skyrocket.

Lub dub, lubdub, lubdub, lubdub, faster and faster and faster, boom, boom, boom, boom, POW! What was that? It nearly threw me to the floor. POW! again. It threw me to the bed. POW! What was this pain, this devil, this evil tormentor in my chest? . . . and then it stopped. Finally it dawned on me that my defibrillator had gone off.

My heart had slowed a bit, but it was still racing nonetheless. We called 911 and my neighbor Nancy, who made the first of her many mid-night visits. As the paramedics struggled to get IVs in me, I felt myself slipping away. "I'm going now"—but no, BAM! again. A stretch of calm, into the ambulance. BAM! BAM! Calm again. BAM! Which of us raced faster, the ambulance or my heart? BAM! Make it stop! Make it stop! BAM!

In all I was shocked sixteen times on the way to the hospital. Shocked into submission. I found myself begging for amiodarone.

I spent several days in the hospital, while they began my drug therapy. The amiodarone did help. My heart rhythm was normal, and I went back home. But within a week I was back in the hospital. The amiodarone wasn't working; indeed it was making things worse, poisoning me and sending my heart into ventricular tachycardia. But what options did I have left? This, as far as I knew, was the only medication that showed any promise of regulating my heart rhythm. These were days of sorrow and fear. The reality of my mortality loomed large. I needed to say good-bye. I wrote to David and Paul.

———— ∽ ————

Life and death have taken on new meanings today. I have had to come to peace with my dying.

My peace comes in knowing that you and Paul have each other. You love each other so much.

My peace comes in knowing such deep love for you and from you, my sweet David. That is the meaning of life and in that I have lived knowing all the fullness of life.

Oh sweet one, I don't want to leave you. I feel we have so much to grow on. I have so much to live for—you, Paul, my work, my family and friends, my rediscovered joy in life.

I have hope—such deep hope for us. How I long to grow old loving you.

There may be difficult choices ahead. I may be institutionalized for months. I may be stabilized and be able to come home. And I may be waiting for a new heart and all that entails.

All I know is that I want nothing more than making a home with you and our sweet baby.

Every moment that we have is precious.

TO DAVID, JUNE 3, 1990

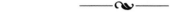

My sweet baby,

It is a day of great sorrow. It is a day I am learning to let go. I have so wanted to live—and I still do with all of my heart—but I also need to reconcile myself to the possibility I may not be around for you much longer.

As I write this, I want you to know that I am always here for you. I can't pick you up and comfort you, or dance around the living room with you, or walk in the woods with you, or watch you discover all the new things in the world, or give you your bath, or rock you to sleep and then greet you in the morning.

But I can love you, always.

I need you to know that you have given me the most wonderful, joyous, miraculous year of my life. You are my sweet angel.

And in this moment when I wonder if I may leave you soon, I feel such gratitude for knowing you, my sweet son. I cherish you.

Still you come to the hospital and cuddle up and read books and sing songs, and I feel the love pour out.

Always know, my sweet Paul, how very loved you are—always.

TO PAUL, JUNE 3, 1990

My doctors put me on a new medication, Rythmol. It had a nice sound to it—more peaceful, more rhythmic than amiodarone. My heart responded well. It was so steady; it almost seemed like a miracle. Then three days later the rhythm worsened again with a string of premature ventricular contractions (PVCs), and my heart was off to the races again. "Bolus of Inderal!" ordered my doctor. When this new medication reached my heart, it slowed to a normal pace. Crisis averted. My wise doctor, who had met me only two weeks before, had figured me out by then. The panic triggered by the PVCs sent my adrenaline shooting up, which made my heart go faster. The Inderal blocked the adrenaline from having its effect on my heart. So in conjunction with the Rythmol, I began regular Inderal therapy. Life was possible. I went home.

My sister, Jeannie, had come from Ohio to care for me and my family, so I focused on healing. I went regularly to cardiac rehab, and the rehab team was excited about my rapid progress. I was walking and biking and rowing farther and faster each time. I began to hope that I could lead a normal life. Then it all turned sour. I began having runs of PVCs and would need to quit my exercises before I got through the session. Eventually the rehab team just stopped trying.

Then began a long saga of trying different medications and different dosages, making trips in and out of the emergency room, stability, and instability. I was fairly incapacitated, especially by fear. In the morning, my heart would beat steadily, by afternoon the rhythm would be bumpy, by evening . . . well, let's just say I could hardly get through a night without dysrhythmia becoming so severe that I wondered whether this night would be my last night. I lived on the edge. My journal entries during the next few months reflect my fears.

I don't know what's ahead for us. It seems just as things are getting stable, they become unsettled again. How I wish I could give you a life filled with happiness and free of cares. . . .

Sometimes I feel like we have all the time in the world. Sometimes, like now, it seems our time together will end far too soon.

TO DAVID, JULY 16, 1990

7

My sweet David,
You are so sad.
Today feels more hopeless. The end feels more inevitable.

TO DAVID, SEPTEMBER 12, 1990

———— ❧ ————

My sweet baby Paul,
I hear you say "bye-bye" as you leave the room and I won-
der if those are the last sounds I will hear from you. That sweet
"bye-bye."

TO PAUL, SEPTEMBER 12, 1990

Over the next several months, as my doctor adjusted the medica-tion dosages, my body seemed to be adjusting too. I think that my heart, made irritable the previous spring by the cardiac arrest, the op-eration to implant the defibrillator, and all the shocks, was gradually healing. By December, seven months after the arrest, I seemed to hit a fairly stable plateau. I rejoined life. We traveled to Michigan for a big Christmas family reunion. During January and February, I enjoyed my days with Paul; I was back in rehab and exercising hard; I found myself getting involved in public debates about the Gulf War and the building of a marina on the shore of Lake Superior near Duluth. So, on a night in mid-February, I once again kissed my husband and baby boy good-bye and this time went off to speak at a public forum on the marina.

———— ❧ ————

I remember walking out of the house that night, giving
you a big hug. If I'd known what lay in store I never would
have walked out that door.

TO PAUL, FEBRUARY 24, 1992

"Is this a bad joke?" I asked my husband, as I awoke once again in a hospital bed, connected to all kinds of wires and tubes and machines and IVs, with some sense that I had done it again. Yes, indeed, I had arrested again, this time while speaking out against the marina project. As with my first arrest, I had no memory of the event, but later was told I'd gone into ventricular tachycardia as I spoke and was shocked repeatedly by my defibrillator before lapsing into unconsciousness. Again, a doctor and nurse in the audience kept me alive with CPR until paramedics arrived. The paramedics fought for over half an hour to stabilize my heart rhythm. They shocked me, my defibrillator shocked me, they pumped me with lidocaine and pumped on my chest, breathing for me and pumping my blood with their own bodies. As I think of it now, it's a major miracle that I survived yet another arrest with my brain intact. One of my greatest fears throughout this whole ordeal was that I would survive an arrest but would be cut off from oxygen for so long that I would have little brain function left and would linger for years in a vegetative state.

But I had escaped again. My heart rhythm stabilized in a few days, and I was once again sent to the University Hospital, where doctors adjusted the settings on my defibrillator. The doctors again began to talk of a heart transplant, but I wouldn't hear of it.

I just wanted to get back home, and home I went.

But I returned home with new questions. I am a university professor, and by chance and good fortune I had previously scheduled a sabbatical for the past year; but in a few months, I would need to be back in the classroom. Could I teach? After my cardiac arrest at the coffeehouse, I no longer felt safe performing music in public. This time, my heart had arrested while I was speaking in public. Well, speaking in public was my job. Granted, the classroom is usually less impassioned than a public forum, but not always. My doctor and I started talking about disability. Disability. What an awful word. I didn't want it. I didn't want to give in to that. I wept at the thought.

My doctor and I also began talking about "next time"—the next time I went into ventricular tachycardia, that is. Since the defibrillator had been implanted in my body, I had experienced two episodes of life-threatening tachycardia, and both times the defibrillator's shocks had failed to convert my heart rhythm. Was the third time the charm, or would I strike out? Next time, I might not be so lucky as to have doctors and nurses around. Next time, I might die. Next time, I might be shocked so many times that I would simply die from the fatigue of it. Next time, I might end up a vegetable. Next time . . . I pondered it in my journal.

———— ❧ ————

It has been a sobering day.

I see this fine line on which I live too clearly today. Most of the time I simply live, trying not to think of my realities, but today I had to think and talk realistically about my disability and about "the next time." "The next time . . ." in which I will either be converted by this device or face a heart transplant or die. I am so well, so alive, with so much to live for . . . and I could be dead any minute.

I suppose I should be glad for this opportunity to live as though each moment were my last, but I tire of the intensity of that. Perhaps the lesson in that is not to live as though death were imminent, but rather to live as though I had a full life ahead of me—and thus it will become full.

When I was a little girl, Mr. Infield would take Kay and me to the circus each year. I would get so tense during the high-wire act. They performed without a net and I would become so anxious that one of them would fall. I just hated it.

Now I feel like I'm walking a tightrope, doing a high-wire act. There is a net beneath me, but it's full of large, gaping holes. I'm trying to stay balanced up here, but should I fall . . .

MARCH 26, 1991

I continued to walk a tightrope, for my heart rhythm never really recovered the stability it had prior to this latest arrest. Without warning, for unknown reasons, even while I was simply lying in bed, it would slip into tachycardia—not fast enough to set off my defibrillator, but terrifying all the same. Dying seemed an imminent possibility.

———— ∾ ————

One of the most baffling aspects of all this is that one of these times, I simply might not wake up. I have always come to, and my life has gone on. What does it mean not to wake up, not to continue, simply to end? That seems an incredible thing to me.

So many of my loved ones' lives have ended. I know what it is to experience the end of another's life. But what would it be simply not to wake up myself? I can't fathom it. . . .

How horrible not to wake up again. Never again to hold my sweet baby or my sweet David in my arms. Never again to hear their laughter or to comfort their tears. Never again to see the sun shining through the leaves or the moonlight on the lake. Not to see Paul as he grows and changes. Not to show him daily my love for him.

I want to go on and on and on.

APRIL 12, 1991

Perhaps it was that strong desire to go on that sustained me through what was to come a few weeks later on a day in early June.

My heart rhythm had been erratic all day—sometimes galloping, other times limping along at an unsteady gait, wobbly, hobbled. I knew that if I went to the emergency room to have it checked, I would end up in the hospital once again—and I couldn't face leaving my little boy for yet another hospital stay. I assured myself that if I stayed home, denying the impending crisis, it would go away. Ignore it long enough, and the bad spell would dissipate.

I went about my day as usual. I was in the midst of heavy planting. We were landscaping our yard made barren from repair and remodeling backhoes. That particular night I was planting daylilies on the side hill. Digging in this dirt is an experience at excavation. If you can chisel your way through the cement of dry clay, you are likely to be stopped at every stab of the shovel by a rock, large or small. It is not an easy task to plant any flower in this soil, let alone ones that need to be planted one inch wide and seven inches deep. It required all my effort. Nevertheless, I had successfully installed about a dozen daylilies and was just finishing planting the last when Paul came to the window fresh from his bath, calling, "Mommy, come in." He wanted me to come in for his bedtime. I wanted to finish planting. I have often wondered how that day might have gone differently if I had heeded his call.

"Just a minute, sweetie. I just want to finish planting this last flower."

"Mommy, come in."

Mommy, come in. That cry haunted me for days afterward. For as I dug, I was vaguely aware that my breathing was heavier, harder. There was sense of apprehension in my chest. And as I climbed the hill to get the watering can, I could no longer ignore the racing of my heart. What was my pulse? 100? 120? My defibrillator was set to go off when my pulse reached 135.

I screamed for David. What should I do? Sit down? Go in the house? That meant climbing stairs. Would that make my heart beat faster?

"David!"

I opted for the house. The pounding came harder and faster. David dialed 911 and then called Nancy. Faster and faster, kaboom, kaboom, kaboom. Aaaauuuuuu . . .

I screamed as my whole body jolted in the pain of electricity searing through my veins my head my neck my stomach my heart. I am choking on sweat on the pit in my stomach oh the pain oh so much pain. And still my heart doesn't stop. It speeds faster, faster, faster, no, no, oh no, here it comes again, oh no, Aauuuoooh! And still it races. Again oh no it's coming again. Oh God, make it stop make it stop make it stop. Make it stop.

With every shock I screamed. With each scream Paul cried. I could hear him in the back bedroom. My baby. My baby. How can I comfort you in this?

By this time Nancy had come. Nancy, my angel of mercy, tried to calm me and keep me safe until the ambulance arrived. But here it comes again. Oh no, faster, faster, faster, POW. Oh God, I am so tired. Make it stop. Please make it stop. Over and over I plead. Over and over I am picked up, knocked down, knocked out, rolled over, hit again and again and again and again. Beat up from the inside out. Over and over it jolts me. The exhaustion overwhelms me. I hear sirens in the background. They give me hope to hang on—and then they fade away. They've lost their way. Oh please hurry. Oh God, here it comes again. Kaboom, kaboom, kaboom, POW! Aaaauuuugh! Oh God, please, please, please . . .

Nancy holds my hand. She keeps me here. I want to fade away. When will it stop?

Finally the ambulance arrives. Either it is the relief of knowing help is near, or the sheer fatigue, or a combination of both, but finally the rhythm converts. It is over. The shocks stop, for now.

Hospitalized again, I spent yet another week away from my baby boy. I had missed so much of his young life, and the separation tore at my heart more than any shocks could.

My sweet Pauly,
I love you so much.
I can hardly stand this separation. I want to be home with you. How I cherish our moments together.
How I long to rock you to sleep, to hold you in my arms, to hear you say "Mommy come." I want to come home and be your mommy.

TO PAUL, JUNE 6, 1991

But I didn't know if I would be home soon. I didn't know if I would ever come home again. Again I wrote my good-byes to my husband.

I feel I am going to leave you soon. This big little heart feels pushed to its limit.

I just want you to know all you have given me—the most beautiful gifts in the world—your incredible love—our deep closeness—this beautiful little boy.

Cherish him, David.

I know that in the days and years ahead when you are left to take care of him alone, you will be tired, angry, frustrated. But cherish every moment. It fleets away so quickly.

I can leave peacefully knowing I am leaving him in such loving hands. And I can leave you more peacefully knowing that you have each other.

And whenever you see the tenderness in his eyes, know that is my love looking through, for he is the child of our love.

Thank you for loving me, for sharing this brief bit of life with me, for holding me through all of this. . . .

Oh, I don't want to leave you. I want to grow old with you. I pray for that chance, but if I am not so blessed, please know you are always my sweet David.

I love you so.

TO DAVID, JUNE 6, 1991

I was certain that the medication I was on, Rythmol, was now having a deleterious effect on my heart rhythm. At my insistence, my doctor took me off the Rythmol and put me on a different medication, but it wasn't very effective. My heart rhythm was still fairly unstable, and I was scared to go home. It seemed that each time I was shocked I lost more of my confidence, my strength, my will to go on. This last time was particularly devastating, perhaps because, unlike my arrests, of which I had no conscious recall, the memory of this latest siege of repeated shocks was so vivid in my mind. I couldn't shake it. I would awake with a jolt in the middle of the night, certain I had been shocked again. In the grocery store, in the halls of the university where I worked, at the beach, I would suddenly see the flash or feel a jolt. My past invaded my present, as it did my future. I kept wondering, when will the shocking come again? I carried the question in my mind and my body and my spirit. When will it come again? I felt like I was living in a mine field, never knowing when I was going to explode. The days were filled with dread.

I was ready for this to stop.

My doctors in Minneapolis had said that if I was shocked repeatedly again, it would be time to talk transplant. Well, I was finally ready, but they weren't. We had a conference with them that left me thinking they believed this was all in my mind. Of course the defibrillator would work, they said. Of course the defibrillator would work? It hadn't in my experience of it. Who was the one not in touch with reality here?

I wrote a long letter to one of the clinic doctors, explaining my situation.

———— ❧ ————

After my cardiac arrest in February, you told my doctor that if things did not go perfectly the next time, then it would be time to talk transplant. I do not consider being shocked eleven times as things going perfectly. Being shocked eleven times indicates to me that my heart responds poorly, at best, to the shocks, and that I cannot rely on the protection of the device.

Since my cardiac arrest in February, I have lived in both fear and hope of "the next event." I knew that either I would be shocked once or twice and converted, which is quite livable; or I would die; or I would live to be able to pursue the transplant route. That event having occurred, having lived through it, I am ready, indeed eager, to pursue the transplant route. Instead I find that door closed to me, waiting once more to see if I survive another event.

I know you have expressed your certainty that my heart would respond well to the defibrillator, but this has not been my experience. I have had three "events," two in which my heart failed to respond to the defibrillator, and one in which it responded poorly at best. I find myself wondering how much my heart can endure. You say that the only gauge you have is shocks. How many more times do I need to be shocked? . . . My

15

concern here is that by the time my nonstandard case fits the standard criteria for a transplant, it will simply be too late.

FROM A LETTER TO MY DOCTOR, JULY 30, 1991

Mercifully, and it felt like such mercy, the doctors reassessed my situation and agreed that the transplant was the best solution for me. In January of 1992, after waiting six months for the insurance company to approve the procedure, I went through four days of rigorous testing of my body and my mind to be sure I was a fit candidate for the transplant. I "passed," and the way was clear. Now the wait began. Now I had hope . . . and fear.

Outwardly, I was leading a fairly normal life. I had returned to work teaching political philosophy at the University of Minnesota-Duluth, where I had graciously been given smaller classes, and I was going through all the typical dilemmas and delights of raising a two-year-old. Inwardly, and in the private spaces of my life, I was often in turmoil—the turmoil of the disease with its disruptions, disabilities, and demands, and the turmoil of my own indecision. I vacillated on my decision to have a transplant so many times. My heart rhythm varied quite a bit. When it got bad, I hoped for the transplant immediately. When it stabilized, I hoped that the wait would be long because the good health offered by the transplant had a life span of its own—five years, maybe ten—and the longer I could put it off, the longer my life might be. During the good times, the normalcy of my life was deceptive, even to me, and I was often lured into thinking I was fine.

———— ❧ ————

I feel so well, the thought of cutting out my heart seems senseless. I know there have been so many times I thought I wouldn't make it through the day, let alone the year. Right now, I feel I could live out a normal life span. . . .

OCTOBER 10, 1992

And yet so many times I wondered if I would make it through the night.

———❦———

I have not felt this despondent for some time. My heart rhythm has been bad for nearly two weeks. My medication level was low, which accounts for this, but even the increased dose hasn't helped. My body just seems to throw it out. For the first time in a long time I am questioning whether I will make it the year and a half before I can get a new heart.

DECEMBER 1, 1991

Every day, whether good or bad, felt like a nightmare from which there was no waking up.

———❦———

I am so tired of this shadow that follows me. I can duck it during the day, but especially any time I awaken, it is there. I have this vague, uneasy feeling that something is wrong, and I have to think for a moment of what it is—then I remember, my heart. This death sentence that hangs over me.

FEBRUARY 5, 1993

The transplant offered me an escape from that death sentence, but it was a reprieve at best. Would it give me five years? Ten? A bittersweet gift to a forty-year-old woman with a four-year-old son.

———❦———

I've been thinking a lot lately about dying young. I can't seem to get the thought out of the back of my mind. Even looking at twenty more years—it's simply not enough time. I find myself wondering if this is what it's like for people in their sixties, or if one comes to a greater acceptance by then. Somehow I don't think so. There will always be so much to learn, to do, to love.

I find myself reading the obituaries and just looking at the ages. I am particularly interested, strangely comforted and yet saddened by the few who die in their thirties and forties. It is as if I feel some camaraderie, some shared sorrow and plight. I feel the deep tragedy and parents' grief for the death of infants. And I feel a vague envy for the people who live well into their eighties and nineties. I envy their time. If I am insatiable for anything it is that.

DECEMBER 3, 1992

It was so strange to be forty years old and so near to my dying. Most of my forty-something friends were busy with their work, their families, planning their futures, while I was planning my funeral. Many of them were in the throes of finding themselves in midlife. Being so near to the end of mine, I envied them their midlife. I really had no one with whom to share this particular point in life's journey.

———— ❧ ————

I feel so alone. I want to talk with someone, but I don't know who. Who can walk this with me? Who can know what it is to have so little time?

My sweet child. I want to be here for all of your growing up. You are so beautiful, so happy, so full of life.

I go around in this cocoon of normalcy, talking about the future as if it might happen. And then something comes up to make me face my mortality. The reality of that is almost too much to bear.

There is just no one I can go to with this, and I am so alone.

APRIL 29, 1993

No matter how I tried to find my peace with all of this, the fact was, I didn't want this. I didn't want any of it.

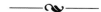

Every once in awhile the revolt will come so strongly upon me. I don't want a transplant. I don't want to live like this. I simply don't want it to be.

SEPTEMBER 19, 1992

In the summer of 1993, the battery on my defibrillator was wearing out, and I needed an operation to replace the old defibrillator with a new one. I had already been waiting a year and a half for a donor heart, and I had hoped a new heart would come before this operation became necessary. The operation seemed so useless. Since the first defibrillator hadn't worked, why bother to put in a new one, even if it was a new, improved model? It was conceivable that my new heart would come the day or the week after the implant surgery, so what was the point of all that pain and expense? But my concerns went beyond these practical issues: I simply didn't know if I would survive the operation.

But I did. All nine hours of it. The doctor tried to locate all the irritable spots in my heart to see whether or not I was a candidate for a new therapy in which those spots were removed. He got to the point where he lost count. Beyond that, the new defibrillator did not work as smoothly as he had hoped. At the end of the surgery, my doctor admitted I might well be part of that 5 percent for whom defibrillators don't work.

I survived the operation, but like the first, it weakened me and made my heart irritable. As I lay in bed one morning just a week after the surgery, my heart once again slipped into tachycardia. Faster, faster, faster, boom, boom, boom . . . I was alone, with Paul asleep in the other room. Faster, faster, boom, boom . . . what to do? I called 911 and Nancy (what would I have done without that woman?), and she arrived just as I was saying, "It's coming. It's coming!" Faster, faster, boom, boom, boom, boom, BAM! I screamed, but this time one shock stopped the tachycardia. By then the paramedics had arrived. David had returned from walking the dog. Paul was awake, but mercifully had missed witnessing this episode. Still, he was visibly shaken. He didn't want me to go, but I was off to the hospital again. Looking out the back ambulance window, watching my life go by once more, I thought for sure that now they would put me to the top of the list and I would get my heart. Let this be the end of it.

But no. After all, the defibrillator had converted my heart with one shock. I could now rest assured that it could and did work for me. Perhaps I should have felt more secure, but I didn't. Now I no longer felt safe anywhere. I had been under the illusion that as long as I did nothing to raise my adrenaline level, I would be safe. So for months I had done nothing that would endanger my life—no fast walking, no digging in the garden, no public speaking, no scary movies. But this last time, I had gone into tachycardia lying in bed. No place was safe. I felt vulnerable to the shocking and to death—anytime, anywhere. I carried the fear all the time, everywhere.

> *What a change a day can make. A week ago my heart went totally out of control and I got shocked again. Now I am afraid to be alone, afraid to go out of the house, afraid to walk— afraid. . . .*
>
> *I want David with me all the time. Or Nancy. That's when I feel most secure.*
>
> *I'm afraid of the fear—that terror as I listen to my heart pound and wait. This is the worst.*
>
> AUGUST 11, 1993

And it wasn't just my fear that concerned me, but Paul's.

> *This is a difficult time for all of us. Last night you were telling me you didn't want the ambulance men to come in the middle of the night. You wanted to be sure I would be there when you woke up in the morning. I wonder what goes on in your head and your heart. Is this always gnawing at the back of your mind as it is mine?*

Nothing's right anymore.

TO PAUL, AUGUST 19, 1993

Over the next few weeks, my heart's condition worsened. The sinus node, which controls the heart's rhythm, was deteriorating, and my pulse often jumped from its normal rate of fifty up to eighty for no discernible reason. When my pulse rate reached one hundred, I would be shocked. At night, the rhythm was so bad I couldn't sleep. The PVCs came in couplets, triplets, quadruplets, sometimes in runs of six and seven. It seemed just a matter of time and luck until I was shocked again . . . or died.

———❧———

I am scared. I am very scared. For weeks I have been focused on the choking confinement of my life, likening it to being on house arrest—let out only to go to work and back. I have been angry and frustrated with my inability to live the way I want to.

But now I am scared. The rhythm is so bad. The EKG showed, as I suspected, that I am having couplets and triplets and sometimes runs of four and five. It seems only a matter of time till one of those runs breaks out. And then will the pacer work? Will the defibrillator work?

The tenuousness of my life is at the center of my focus— perhaps magnified. I just wish the phone call would come soon. I worry it will not come in time.

OCTOBER 12, 1993

Just when I thought this couldn't get much worse, it did. On a night in early November of 1993, I awoke in the middle of the night feeling odd, like I had a horrible, horrible case of the flu. I just couldn't move. I just couldn't . . . I couldn't. I really couldn't. I couldn't lift my head, move my arm, roll over.

"David!" I cried out in a loud whisper. "Something is terribly,

terribly wrong. Something is terribly, terribly wrong. I can't move. Call Nancy."

By that time I was lucid enough to realize I was probably having a stroke. I had been through lots of scary things, but this was the most frightening. What if I were never able to move again? What did this mean for the hope of a transplant? Would they call it off? What did this mean for my life? Even if I got a new heart, would I ever walk again? Write? Hold my baby? Would I live my life in a wheelchair?

The feeling and movement slowly returned to my left side. By the time Nancy arrived, my left side was back to normal and my right side, though weak, was movable. She had me try to lift my right arm and leg. It was as if huge weights were attached to them. With all my might, I could barely lift them, but they did move.

With that, and the fact I could talk, she felt assured I would be okay. She thought it best just to go back to sleep and see how I was in the morning. I was scared, but somehow managed to get back to sleep. In the morning, I had definite weakness on my right side; my legs buckled under me a few times as I walked, but I could walk; I could move my arms. I could move! What a feeling of relief, but also insecurity. Why did this happen? And would it happen again?

An echocardiogram revealed a blood clot in my left ventricle. My doctors assumed that part of the clot had broken off and temporarily closed off an artery in my brain. Luckily the clot was small enough to pass through. They put me on blood thinners and said I would be out of danger from this and future blood clots in about a week.

That was a very long week—the fears gnawing in the back of my mind, wondering if the clot would move from my heart to my brain. Wondering if I would lose my sight, my speech, my ability to walk. In many ways, this was the scariest chapter of all. I have such deep respect for those who suffer strokes or accidents that leave their faculties or their limbs impaired, and who go on. I didn't know if I had the strength to endure that, and perhaps that's why I was spared.

This episode brought an added dimension of fear to my life. Even after I felt fairly protected by the Coumadin (a blood-thinning medication), I would sometimes be afraid to go to sleep, the memory of waking up paralyzed still strongly with me. This more than anything made the decision for the transplant feel right. It wasn't just a rhythm problem anymore. My heart was putting me at risk in other ways as well.

It was putting my family at risk too. They say that illnesses often take more of a toll on the caretakers than the patients. David got pneumonia. Now it was my turn to take care of him and Paul and myself. I needed to get better, and by some grace I did. The rhythm stabilized. Again I was asking myself if I needed the transplant.

Christmas 1993. My niece, Olivia, my sister, Jeannie, and her family had all come to visit. Unlike the previous Christmas, which I had spent in and out of the emergency room, I was doing pretty well. Two days after Christmas, I was on the phone with someone when the call-waiting signal came on. It always seemed so rude to ask whomever I was talking with to wait while I answered another call, and it never was the call I was waiting for—the heart. I ignored the call-waiting, but it came again. This time I thought I'd better answer it. Well, I had been wrong. This was the call I'd been waiting for after all. It was time.

I had a mixture of feelings as David and my nephew, Mark, drove me to the airport—anxiety, uncertainty, sadness, hope. On that cold, clear morning the helicopter took me on a journey to a new life. When I got to the hospital, there was flurry of blood tests, throat cultures, prepping for surgery. It was all going so fast. Shouldn't I think about this some more? And then I waited. I lay there a long time waiting for the surgery. I waited there too long waiting for the surgery. Something was wrong. The donor heart wasn't good enough. They sent me home.

I had a "dry run" on Monday. Everyone was here. The weather was good. David, Paul, and I were all well taken care of. The helicopter flight was fun. When we landed, I had this feeling of "I've made it." I got to this without further complications and before I died. There was a moment of "Hallelujah!"

And there was doubt. Was I really making the right choice? There I was at the moment and still unsure.

And then there was the reprieve—and the disappointment. The heart was not good enough. "We want you to be at Paul's college graduation," said Sofia (one of the transplant coordinators). She understands how I view time through the perspective of the years and events in Paul's life.

And so I came home. And cried. I was ready for the waiting and the wondering to be over. In the months and years of waiting, never have I felt the heaviness of this so much as at this time.

JANUARY 2, 1994

Now the waiting and the indecision began in earnest. By mid-February, I was in my deepest period of doubt. I had been asked to participate in a study for an experimental antirejection drug after the transplant. Going over the consent form, which elaborated on all that could go wrong with a transplant, all my fears surfaced.

——— ❧ ———

The consent form reminded me of all the possible complications of the transplant, and I have felt sucked into the negativity. I think of the transplant and I conjure up AIDS and cancer and glaucoma and osteoporosis and kidney failure and CMV and some massive virus or infection that will take me before I've even had a chance to live again.

FEBRUARY 23, 1994

Rejection, infection, cancer, AIDS . . . I didn't want to risk any of it. This life was good enough. I began rethinking my decision. I called my sister. I called transplant recipients. All confirmed that I needed to go ahead. Still, I questioned. On February 23, I wrote a long letter to Sofia and Sue, the transplant coordinators, asking all kinds of questions. Was this the right thing to do? That night I wrote in my journal:

———— ∞ ————

Here I am in a quandary again. . . .

"The point is to live the questions" (Rilke). Well, I've been living the questions for years now. And perhaps the point is we never really know the answers.

But I wish this were clearer.

These long periods of stability confuse me—lull me into a false (?) sense of safety and normalcy. On these days when I am feeling so well and being productive and pushing myself just a little farther—without the slightest grumble or rumble from my heart—the whole proposition of a transplant seems absurd.

When my heart is in a dysrhythmic mode, the reality is so close that it outweighs the negativity of the transplant. When it is calm, the negativity looms large.

I panic. I run. There is nowhere to go. I am trapped inside this body that will never be fully well again, and that may at any moment fail me altogether.

There have been times when my body has been healthy and strong, but my spirit battered, broken, deadened. Now it is my body that is weak and my spirit that is strong. I want my body to rise up with my spirit.

FEBRUARY 23, 1994

On the ten o'clock news that night there was a story about organ donation—not a particularly newsworthy item, mainly filler, but it of course caught my attention; and watching it I felt that yes, indeed, the transplant was the right thing to do. Ten minutes later the phone rang. It was Sofia. Why was she calling so late at night? Oh. Oh! My time for questioning was over. It was time to act.

I tried to wake Paul. I had always told him I would wake him if he was sleeping when the call came, but he would not be roused. So I left him with Nancy, while David drove me to the hospital. As we sat and waited for the helicopter, we were filled with the sense of what a sad time this must be for somebody. Somebody somewhere had just lost a loved one. We waited in a kind of quiet sympathy and respect.

As the helicopter lifted me off again, I gazed back on the lights of this city and the lake that I love, and knew I would not see it again for some time.

This time, it was a good heart.

The operation went well. My husband, my brothers, my nephew all had come, and I remember a feeling of jovial good humor and celebration following the operation. But just moments after they left the room, something felt terribly wrong. I was slipping away. I told the nurses, and indeed, I was bleeding, bleeding profusely into my chest tubes. I knew at that moment that I was very near death. It was all in God's hands now.

God's and the surgeon's. They whisked me back to the operating room and in ten minutes had me under and open. A stitch had slipped in the main aorta, and I was bleeding to death. But they caught it in time, the second operation was successful, and I began the recovery process. One week later I left the hospital to spend the next three months recovering at David's aunt's home near the hospital.

———— ❧ ————

We did it. Here I am in Aunt Betty's house recovering. I have a new heart. It's all really been done. No more dilemmas, no more wondering, no more waiting. Just time to move on with this new life.

I feel like I have a new life inside me—the heart of a nine-year-old child. It is small and fast, but pumps really well. I want to take care of it as if it were a child within my care. I think of all it has been through and want to nurture it through this time of healing. I can't imagine rejecting it—we feel so sympatico.

It has been stopped and started again twice. . . . Now the poor thing is being pumped with so many drugs and pressured by high blood pressure. On Thursday they took four snips of the inside of it (my first biopsy to check for signs of rejection). *I felt as if I were holding it all during the biopsy—telling it we'd get through this together.*

It is good to feel a young strong, reliable heart inside me— one I do not feel may give way at any moment. Yet I miss my old heart. It saw me through so much. It was dissected and examined and is probably nothing but ashes now—but such a road we traveled together. . . .

The immediacy of fear is gone. I am not constantly monitoring my heartbeat—living in fear of tachycardia and shocks. I think I can fully relax for the first time in four years. What an amazing feeling that is . . . I am free.

Thank you.

Thank you to this sweet child, part of whom now continues inside me. I am so sad for the child's family and friends. And I am so grateful for this second chance. I will do all I can to give it my best in every way.

MARCH 6, 1994

My recovery seemed both fast and slow. My days, spent in the clinic or rehabilitation or asleep, went by quickly, but my nights were often long and pain-filled. My mind often seemed blurry, and trying to carry on a conversation was tortuous. I sometimes wondered if I'd ever be able to think straight again. My progress over the next few weeks was steady, but peppered with scares.

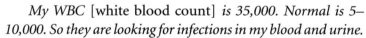

My WBC [white blood count] is 35,000. Normal is 5– 10,000. So they are looking for infections in my blood and urine. So far no word.

MARCH 7, 1994

We have passed through another scare—viral hepatitis. The mention of the possibility threw me into a panic, as I thought of reliving all I had gone through twenty years ago—and perhaps not making it this time. [My initial heart condition was accompanied by hepatitis, and it was suspected that a virus had caused both the hepatitis and the damage to my heart.]

But the ultrasound was normal, so I'm off that particular hook.

MARCH 21, 1994

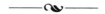

And now I fear pneumonia. I just have a little cold, but I fear the worst. . . . I just don't know what it really means to be immunosuppressed. . . . This is all new.

MARCH 23, 1994

I had the good company of my sister throughout this. She made my meals, walked with me, drove me everywhere I needed to go, spent long hours at the clinic with me, held my hand in my middle of the nightly bouts with pain. Still, the separation from my husband and son often made the time drag so slowly.

I just want so much to go home and be with my family. Poor Paul was so sad today, not being together for his birthday. I need to be home with him. It's just been too long. I don't want anything to delay my homecoming, even for a day.
I need to go home.

MARCH 23, 1994

Gradually, I was getting better, stronger. I could walk a little farther, a little faster. The pain lessened. I had a bit more energy. I could even make it around the grocery store. And then, weeks before I had expected it, they announced to me that I could go home.

———∿———

I'm too excited to sleep. I may be going home next week . . . I may be going home. I just can't imagine anything more wonderful.
MARCH 31, 1994

Home. What a lovely word. What a lovely world. In April of 1994, six weeks after the transplant, not quite four years since this ordeal of a lifetime started, I went home and began my life anew.

In the ensuing months and now years, my life has pretty much returned to normal. I have returned to work. My son has gone on to kindergarten, and now first grade. He is blossoming in the new security and lightness of life in our home. My husband can go off fishing for hours without wondering if I'll be alive when he gets home. I am back to swimming and hiking and dancing. The nightmare of those four years between the cardiac arrest and the transplant seems almost a dream now, though it does come back to haunt me now and again. As I leave the house, I'll find myself running through the checklist of medications to stabilize my heart rhythms, and then remind myself I don't need them anymore; or I'll wake with a start, thinking I've just been shocked; or a movie or an event will trigger a subconscious memory of that time. But mostly it is far from my mind.

I still am tied to antirejection medication and various medical procedures, though not nearly so many as before the transplant. It hasn't been completely smooth sailing, and I have had a few scares along the way. Four months after my transplant, I suffered an episode of rejection. The impending loss of this new heart, and my life, was dreadful. However, a few days of megadoses of IV prednisone stopped the rejection. At the time, I was quite frightened. Now it just seems a little blip, one of the many I'm sure we'll have to deal with.

A couple of times, test results indicated the possibility of cancer, but they turned out to be minor disorders. Other than these, I have been extraordinarily healthy. I've rarely even had a cold.

Though life continues as usual, it will never be the same. How can I ever watch the sunrise without an acute appreciation of the dawning of a new day in my life? How can I ever take a walk without gratitude for that gift so easily taken for granted? How can I run barefoot down the beach and not the feel an extraordinary lightness in my heart? How can I see the sparkle in my son's eyes and not feel a great gladness?

The whole of it—the illness, the despair, the fear, the horror, and the literal waking to a new life filled with gratitude, wonder, and joy—have taken me on quite a journey—two journeys really. The one, my physical life journey through the illness itself is all I have related up to this point. But it is the other journey—a journey of the spirit—a journey of the heart—that has had the larger impact on my life. It is not a journey that I would have wanted or could have planned, but it has taken me where I have needed to go.

In the chapters that follow, I share the insights into patience, hope, gratitude, joy, and love that I was granted along the journey of my spiritual heart.

> *How strange his life had been, he thought.*
> *He had wandered along strange paths. . . .*
> *And yet this path has been good . . .*
> *I have had to experience so much. . . .*
> *just in order to become a child again and begin anew.*
> *But it was right that it should be so;*
> *my eyes and heart acclaim it. . . .*
> *Whither will my path yet lead me? . . .*
> *it goes in spirals, perhaps in circles,*
> *but whichever way it goes,*
> *I will follow it.*

HERMANN HESSE, *Siddartha*

Sick at heart

A new heart I will give you, and a new spirit
I will put within you; and I will take out of your flesh
the heart of stone and give you a heart of flesh.

EZEKIEL 36:26

Much of what I endured, others with serious or life-threatening illness have also endured. Much of what I learned has been learned by transplant recipients who received other organs—a liver, kidney, pancreas, or lung. But it was of particular significance to me that it was my heart that was sick.

The heart is so central to our identity, our self, our soul. It is at the core of our very being. It is the pulse of our life. Its connections with love and compassion, with courage and sincerity, are wrapped deep in our language and our culture. To "hearten" is to encourage. We "take heart," and we "lose heart." When we are fully engaged in a belief or a task, we are "wholehearted," and when not, we are only "halfhearted," or "our heart's not in it" at all. When we want to be clear about what we are feeling about something, we "search our hearts." When we speak our deepest feelings we "pour our hearts out." When something affects us deeply and sincerely we "take it to heart." When we feel a close affinity with someone we say they are "after our own hearts." When we bring our emotions to the surface we "wear our hearts on our sleeve." When we feel tenderness, it "warms our heart," and when we feel sympathy it pulls at our "heartstrings." When we grieve we feel "heartache," and the loss of love renders us "heartbroken." We can be "bighearted," "tenderhearted," "heavyhearted," "lighthearted," "softhearted," "hardhearted," or totally "heartless."

Hearts are everywhere, in symbol and saying. Over the past few years, every card my sister sends me has a saying about a heart on it. The calendar she got me for one of my years of waiting was called "Feelings of the Heart" and was filled with expressions like "Listen to your heart, to the messages it sends you." Over the years she has given me a heart blanket, a heart rug, a heart T-shirt, a heart poster, a heart key chain, and a rattan heart to hang on the wall. My son has joined in and makes me pictures of hearts, construction-paper hearts, and hearts made of Play-Doh. Even the U.S. Post Office has gotten into it; most of the cards sent to me after my transplant had heart stamps on them. At my heartwarming party (to celebrate my new heart), people brought me heart candles, heart suckers, even artichoke hearts and hearts of palm. The heart is pervasive in our culture, in a way that lungs, livers, and kidneys are not. (Well, I suppose there are kidney beans.)

And the heart holds meaning in a way that other organs do not. In our culture, we particularly link hearts with love. On Valentine's Day, we give hearts. The Tin Man went to the Wizard of Oz in search of a heart, so he could love again. Indeed, the heart has become a kind of shorthand symbol for the word *love*. We find it on T-shirts and mugs and bumper stickers—"I ❤ golden retrievers" or "I ❤ golf" or "I ❤ America."

Beyond language and popular culture, the heart is a touchstone of so many spiritual traditions. In Buddhism, the path of compassion, of loving kindness, of spiritual rightness, is the "path with heart." In Hinduism, the heart is the center of seven chakras, or spiritual energy centers, the one that is the seat of love. The heart is ubiquitous in the Judeo-Christian tradition. According to the concordance, there are nearly seven hundred references to the "heart" in the Bible alone (and that's only the singular; there's another classification for "hearts"). And try to get through a worship service without mention of the heart. Even if not mentioned in the invocation, the benediction, or the pastoral prayers, it's bound to come up in the hymns. One is hard-pressed to find a hymn without it.

Rejoice, ye pure in heart

Hearts unfold like flowers before thee

Now thank we all our God, with heart and hand and voices

Spirit of God descend upon my heart

The list goes on . . .

In the Bible, the heart is often referred to as the seat of joy, thankfulness, compassion, integrity, sincerity, courage, purity, righteousness. For example:

Thou has put more joy in my heart than they have when their grain and wine abound.—Psalm 4:7

A glad heart makes a cheerful countenance.—Proverbs 15:13

My words declare the uprightness of my heart.—Job 33:3

Create in me a clean heart, O God.—Psalm 51:10

*His heart was courageous in the ways of the Lord.
—2 Chronicles 17:6*

Blessed are the pure in heart.—Matthew 5:8

*My heart is steadfast, O God, my heart is steadfast!
—Psalm 57:7*

And the greatest commandment is:

*Hear, O Israel: The Lord our God is one Lord; and you shall love the Lord your God with all your heart, and with all your soul, and with all your might. And these words which I command you this day shall be upon your heart.
—Deuteronomy 6:4–6*

The heart also seems to be the seat of sin and temptation, especially for the sin of pride.

Haughty eyes and a proud heart, the lamp of the wicked, are sin.—Proverbs 21:4

And the heart which is not strong may be the place of fear and failure. For evils have encompassed me without number; my iniquities have overtaken me, till I cannot see; they are more than the hairs of my head; my heart fails me.—Psalm 40:12

I asked myself how I had failed to be loving, courageous, pure, righteous? My spiritual journey began by plunging into the heart of darkness—of judgment and blame—of seeing a literal connection between the failings of my physical heart and the failings of my spiritual heart.

Perhaps it was wrong to look for any kind of literal meaning in my illness. After all, the heart is just another organ, like the liver, gall bladder, and spleen. But I was so surrounded, sometimes bombarded, by the language, the symbol, the meaning, how could I not? And though I recognize the very real part played by viruses, bacteria, and injury, I do believe we can and do become diseased, in part, from the afflictions of our minds and hearts and spirits, which settle in particular places in our bodies.

I was encouraged in this belief by the New Age movement of self-healing, which embraces the body-mind connection and encourages one to look to the location of the illness to understand its true source in one's life, thereby coming to a direction for healing. For example, in her *You Can Heal Your Life*, Louise Hay presents a list to which one can refer to get a sense of one's illness from its physical location in the body. One can simply look up the affected organ for a quick diagnosis of the problem. Under "Heart" one finds:

Heart—represents the center of love and security

Problems: long-standing emotional problems. Lack of joy. Hardening of the heart. Belief in strain and stress.

In their book *The Creation of Health,* Norman Shealy and Caroline Myss analyze the energy factors associated with illness, and conclude this about heart disease:

We are, by nature, a tribal species. We need each other and we need to be needed by each other. We need to give love as well as receive love. We thrive when we are loved and we are diminished in strength and vitality without love.

Yet in spite of the simplicity of our needs, we remain deeply confused about the nature of love. It seems that we have separated our natural capacity to love and be loving from the activity of living. Most, if not all, of us exist somewhere between the simplicity of our needs and the complexity of our fears and insecurities that share the space of our hearts. . . .

. . . We need to begin with evaluating what is preventing the natural flow of love through each person's life. . . .

Broken hearts are real. Every human being has his or her limits when it comes to absorbing grief, hurt, rejection and despair. . . .There comes a point at which a person is incapable of "getting up again," of trying one more time to recover from the loss or absence of love in one's life. This is the crisis of a broken heart, and . . . it can stop the heart completely.

NORMAN SHEALY and CAROLINE MYSS, *The Creation of Health*

All this rang true for me. In the decade preceding my 1990 cardiac arrest, I had gone through a very difficult period of grief and loss—the dissolution of my first marriage, the deaths of my parents and one of my dearest friends in life, the deaths of both my dogs, and deeply loved loves that turned sour. My heart had been broken, and my response was to harden it. Sealing myself off from ever again knowing such pain, I had encased my heart from ever loving so deeply again. Even though newly remarried, I felt I was preventing the natural flow of love through my life. Following a session with a therapist who was helping with my healing in that period between the birth of my son and my cardiac arrest a year later, I wrote:

———— ⟋⟍ ————

I was struck by the metaphoric parallel between our talking about my holding back on loving David and the medical descriptions of what is going on with my heart—"backpressure"; the need to "unload" my heart and reduce my blood pressure. It seems I have dammed myself up, in a variety of ways. I have not let myself just flow. I have dammed up my heart—my love, my music, my writing, my movement, my generosity. I need to let all these flow.

I am struck by the image of the stream being dammed. I've let all this debris clog up the stream. As it has clogged, it has created a reservoir behind it—the dilated ventricle. As I start to unclog the debris, the blood will flow more freely and the ventricle return to normal size.

SEPTEMBER 13, 1989

I was convinced that if I could just unclog my emotional heart, my physical heart would heal.

New Age self-healing was not the only tradition to send me looking for the meaning of my illness. Traditional spiritual paths did so as well. In Eastern religions, one's spiritual energies are deeply associated with illness and healing. Chinese spirituality focuses on "chi," the spiritual energy of the universe that flows or is trapped in various parts of our body. Hinduism speaks of this in terms of seven "chakras," or energy centers, through which one's spiritual energy flows. I do very much see my bodymind as an energy system. (I do regard my being as bodymind, finding the mind/body separation to be a false construction of our culture.) It fits with my intuitive sense of myself. And my intuitive sense of myself was that the energy surrounding my heart was blocked. My enlarged heart and rhythm disturbances were also evidence to me that I was blocking the energy to my heart. That the chakra before the heart chakra affects the adrenal gland also struck me deeply. My adrenal gland was overflowing, another sign to me that the energy got blocked at the heart and simply couldn't get through. I had closed off my heart. I needed to open it again. I worked with meditation tapes to open my heart chakra. I did exercises in the Eastern spiritual practices of tai chi and chi gong, both of which work with directing the energy flow in the body, to help release the energy flow in my body. The chi gong was so powerful it sent me into tachycardia, and I had to abandon it.

Throughout my searchings for the meaning of my illness, I carried a sense of shame. The language and the culture and the spiritual traditions were all telling me that I had closed off my heart, hardened my heart, blocked the flow to my loving. What kind of a person would do that?

But what most deeply filled me with shame was the Judeo-Christian tradition in which I had been raised and with which I was surrounded. This tradition led me to regard my illness as a punishment for the crimes of my heart. I had sinned, in a variety of ways, primarily in the failure of my first marriage and in the longings of my heart, and now I was being punished. In the depths of my despair, images of a cruel and mocking God came to me, proclaiming that I would never be happy again. This was a harsh and vengeful God.

How did I come to this? I remember pouring this out to a friend, who became almost angry, asking, "Is that really what you believe of God?" No, intellectually I didn't believe this of God. I had been taught that God was loving and forgiving, but the sense of punishment was so strong. Especially now, now that life was good, with my loving husband and the baby I had hoped for all of my life—to take it all away seemed cruel, tempting, taunting—an act of vengeance.

The Bible is full of images of God using illness, particularly illness of the heart, as a punishment.

> *Your ways and your doings have brought this upon you. This is your doom, and it is bitter; it has reached your very heart.*
>
> JEREMIAH 4:18

> *Thou wilt give them dullness of heart; thy curse will be on them.*
>
> LAMENTATIONS 3:65

The joy of our hearts has ceased;
our dancing has been turned to mourning. . . .
Woe to us, for we have sinned!
For this our heart has become sick. . . .
Art thou exceedingly angry with us?

LAMENTATIONS 5:15–17, 22

Was God exceedingly angry with me? Was I being punished, and for what crimes? What had I done to make God so angry that he—my image of a vengeful God was always of a "he"—made my heart sick? Had I loved too little? Was I not loving enough to my husband, to my child, to my family and friends? My heart was too big. Perhaps I had loved too much? Perhaps I had loved too easily, without thought? Had I loved my heart out?

The commandment to "Love thy neighbor as thyself" came to me. Perhaps the "as thyself" was my failure. Was my sin in being unwilling and unable to love myself? Part of my healing journey took me to a holistic healer/M.D. Shortly into my therapy with him, I had the most powerful dream of my life. Coincidentally (?) I had written in my journal five days before, "I have often had feelings of my need to be punished."

In the dream, I was being prepped for surgery, a standard post-pregnancy operation, in which a thin film was stretched over the brain. A woman came into the operating room looking for me.

She was all hunched over. They pulled her head back so I could see her face and asked me if I knew her. I didn't.

Her eyes were filled with a crazed hate. I have never seen such hate, such despising. She raved on and on about how she'd come to get me and was determined to contaminate the operating field. She started by spitting on everything. Jerry (the doctor) and his assistant tried to grab her to stop her, so she said she'd pee on everything, which she proceeded to do. When they stopped her from doing that, she started vomiting all over. Then she disappeared.

The next thing I remember I was going to a late-night movie. I went into the restroom with a friend to change Paul's diaper. It was the only place I felt safe.

When I returned home—which was an upstairs apartment in a run-down neighborhood—Jerry, who was now a police officer, was conducting a house-to-house search for her.

(I think it was at this point that I remembered that a woman had called my house the day before the operation. My sister answered the phone, and the woman had told her that she was coming to get me.)

I went into my apartment and was trying to lock the door behind me, when I realized someone was pushing on the door to get in. It was the woman. Terrified, I pushed back. She pushed; I pushed.

AUGUST 20, 1989

At that point I woke up, screaming, heart pounding, shaking, sobbing uncontrollably. I was still quite terrified. I was afraid to go back to sleep. The only thing that enabled me to go back to sleep was to return to this woman in my mind, stop running from her, face her, and talk with her with compassion.

The next time I saw my healer, we did a gestalt of the dream. I put myself back in the dream and became the woman. This led me on an incredible journey of reexperiencing my birth. I had been born prematurely, cesarean, because my mother had toxemia and was in danger of losing her life. Indeed, she had often told me that she went into the hospital that day to die. She was critically ill, and when I was born they took me from her and placed me in an incubator. I did not see her for days.

In my rebirthing experience, I was cold, so very cold. I rocked and rocked myself. "Where was she?" I wondered. "I want her. I want her voice, her body, her warmth, her heart beating next to mine. Where is she? Where is she? I'm so cold. I'm so very cold. I must be bad, so bad to make her go away. What did I do?"

What I discovered in this process was that I blamed myself for being born. I blamed myself for my mother being sick, for nearly dying, for being the cause of the debilitating and life-threatening high blood pressure that accompanied her the rest of life. Had I lived in self-blame all of my life? Was my heart failure a failure to love myself? Perhaps this was the source of my illness.

My source of blame was also my source of hope. If I could cause my own illness, then I could also heal myself. However, even though I had discovered the source of my illness, if indeed I had, I still wasn't healing. All the meditating, the tai chi, the chi gong, the self-forgiveness exercises weren't working. I had failed again. My continuing illness was evidence of my failure—my failure to heal. I wasn't good enough, pure enough of heart, faithful enough. I condemned myself all the more.

What finally pulled me out of this pit of self-blame and self-condemnation was Steven Levine's *Healing Into Life and Death*. He at one point talks about how even the world's greatest saints have sickened and died. Perhaps this wasn't a question of punishment. Perhaps this was, as he says,

> *An opportunity to become healed. To discover the true nature of love and the wholeness, the complete spaciousness, of an unhindered awareness, to receive life directly, as it is, with no filters or unfinished business. Just things as they are, just being itself.*

STEPHEN LEVINE, *Healing Into Life and Death*

Rather than asking what is the source of the illness, or how is healing to be done, or even should healing be done, he suggests we ask the question, "Where is healing to be found?" The basic message of his work is that the healing that needs to be done in our lives is a spiritual healing, which may or may not have anything to do with physical healing.

I think of my friend Lucy, who died of cancer several years ago now. I have never been able to see auras, but I saw hers. A few weeks before her death, I visited her in the hospital where she had gone for treatment. She was positively glowing. White light, the color of spiritual awareness, surrounded her. In those last days of physical illness and demise, she was spiritually healed.

Perhaps my illness was presenting me with an opportunity to learn some spiritual lessons I needed to learn. My heart was sick, and I imagine both physiological and psychological factors contributed to that. But I was also sick at heart. I had heart lessons to learn, lessons about love and wonder, compassion and forgiveness, patience and humility, gratitude and joy, that only life could teach me. For many people, these lessons are reserved for the final hours of their life, and perhaps they carry these lessons on with them to another sphere. My miracle and blessing were that I was gifted with both the opportunity to glimpse these insights and the chance to start my life anew—to turn, to live.

> *Cast away from you all the transgressions which you have*
> *committed against me, and get yourselves a new heart and a*
> *new spirit! Why will you die, . . . for I have no pleasure in the*
> *death of any one, says the Lord God; so turn and live.*
>
> EZEKIEL 18:31–32

Letting go and trust

Let it go. Let it go.
This water belongs in Mombasa.

Out of Africa

In this scene from the movie *Out of Africa,* the rains have come, and Karen and the workers are struggling valiantly to keep intact the dam they had built to irrigate the crops. They pile sandbag upon sandbag, but the force of the river is too strong. It keeps breaking through the sandbags until finally Karen says, "Let it go. Let it go. This water belongs in Mombasa."

That image of letting the water go—letting it burst the dam, letting it flow—had, over the years, helped me through countless times when I had wanted to hang on—to old loves, old hurts, past pains, and broken promises. Whenever I caught myself hanging on, I would bring this image to mind. It always helped me to release my grasp. "Let it go. Let it go. This water belongs in Mombasa."

Now I was facing new challenges of letting go. As I wrote in my journal:

———— ❧ ————

It seems I have dammed myself up, in a variety of ways. . . . I need to let all these flow. . . . I need to spend time unclogging the stream—seeing it, hearing it, feeling it. As I flow, so will my heart.

SEPTEMBER 13, 1989

I worked on letting myself flow in my love and my life. I even visualized unclogging the dams around my heart; but it was too little too late. My heart arrested eight months later. However, the cardiac arrest itself seemed to open the floodgates holding back my loving. My journals to my husband and baby boy at the time are filled with the overflowing of my love for them. Certainly the fragility of my life took my husband and me to a deeper phase in our love and commitment to each other.

Little did I know the challenges of letting go that lay ahead. For the rains had come, and the river of my life, as well as each confluent rivulet, had just flooded its banks and burst its dams. I'd been flooded out of my life—swept downstream from my child, my home, my work, my future—and I wanted to grasp at every passing tree and limb. My life was out of control, and I was having a hard time letting it go.

My life was out of control in big ways, but it was the little ways that drove me wild. Those little areas of life we carve out for ourselves—the particularities of our existence that we want just so. Little things, like the laundry. Was it done in cold water or warm? Were the stains removed? How were the shirts folded and the socks rolled up? Little things, like how my car was driven. I was not allowed to drive for six months, so my husband loaned his car to his sister and drove mine instead. He drove it too hard—too fast over the bumps, too jerky on the clutch, too heavy on the brakes. I was quite the backseat driver. I even found it hard to keep my peace about the choice of parking spots. Little things, like how my garden was tended, or how the dishwasher was loaded, or whether the vacuuming got done. I wanted to control them all.

My life was out of control in big ways. Perhaps that's why I clung to the little things.

Then there was Paul. He was out of my control, out of my reach, out of my grasp. All the things I hadn't wanted him exposed to, he was: sugar, he got his first Popsicle; TV, he was watching *Sesame Street*. I had no control over these influences on him. I was no longer in charge of his daily care.

But these were incidental in the overall scheme of things. Two issues about raising a child I had felt so strongly about were stripped from me. One, I had never wanted my child to feel abandoned. I had worked hard to cultivate a sense of security and trust in Paul. Except when asleep in his crib, he spent most of his first few months in a Snugli, attached to one or the other of us as we went about our day. When I went back to work when he was six months old, David stayed home with him. I had never left him for more than a few hours until that night on May 4 when I left him for weeks. This was not how it was supposed to be. To be so tightly bonded—then nothing. How confusing to him, how bewildering, how harsh to wake up that morning and find his morning comfort and milk and mom gone. Oh, this was not what I had wanted at all.

His sense of trust in me was gone. Perhaps, had I not held him so tightly he would have been better prepared. He didn't trust me again for a long time. And that was so harsh. We were estranged.

——— ❧ ———

Dearest Paul,

We are so estranged, you and I, and we love each other so much.

Maybe we were too tightly bonded and we needed this separation in order for you to become your own person.

Tonight I experienced the deep sorrow and pain and loss and bewilderment you must have felt that morning when you woke up and first found me gone—no mama, no milk—everything was different.

Now mama is home and so much is still different. I remember the way I used to twirl you around till we were both so dizzy, and the way I used to pick you up and toss you around, and our long walks—all gone. How strange it must seem to you. You seem to have pulled farther away from me since I've

*come home—perhaps because our relationship is so different
from the time I left. Do you think I am rejecting you?*

*I probably am too intent on bringing back that feeling of
oneness and completeness that we shared. I have never known
anything like it. I miss it so much. I miss us so much.*

Instead, what I feel now is estrangement. . . .

*That is the ache in my heart—the connection is gone. I am
a stranger to you, and you to me.*

TO PAUL, JUNE 30, 1990

He would not come to me for comfort. I would pick him up and hold
him when he cried, and he would push me away and reach for Daddy.

The thing I used to hate about baby-sitting was that the babies
simply could not be comforted. They wanted their mama, and that
wasn't me. Now it was me, and I still couldn't comfort him. How I
ached for him. Maybe he ached for me too. But his sense of trust in
me was broken.

I'd wanted him to feel security—a sense of trust in a benevolent
universe, the loving mother arms—and bemoaned its loss. But what
of me? Was I trusting the universe to hold him? I didn't want to let go.
I needed to let go.

Some trust must have been created in all our time together, for
eventually the dam broke, and he tumbled into my arms once more.

My sweet Paul,

*We seem to have broken through a wall today. We had such
a delightful time together. I'm not sure what we did. I just know
that we were together, really together. You lighten and brighten
my heart.*

*Today we fell in love again. I don't know how or why—
we just finally found each other again. Maybe it was playing
on the slide, or playing keep-away in the yard, or filling up
the watering cans over and over, or walking down the hill*

together—whatever we did today was touched with magic.
How we giggled and laughed.

> *Thank you, my sweet baby, for coming back to me.*
>
> TO PAUL, JULY 9, 1990

Still, this was not the life for him I'd planned. It was a life of fear, a life of chaos. It was not a life I wanted for my child.

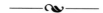

> *I am missing you so much tonight. I only saw you for five minutes today. I wanted hours. I want to be there for you first thing in the morning and last thing at night.*
>
> *It is a month since I have lived day in and day out with you. I had not wanted to leave you, even for a day. Even the hours of the day I had to be away were so hard.*
>
> *This is not how I wanted it to be, sweet one.*
>
> TO PAUL, JUNE 4, 1990

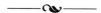

> *Whenever I think of how this summer was supposed to be, I am so sad.*
>
> *Finally we would have day upon day upon day to be together*
>
> *to go for walks in the woods*
> *to go to the beach*
> *to swirl you through the water naked and watch you giggle with delight*
> *to explore all the new flowers and grasses and bugs*
> *to throw stones in the lake*
> *for all of us to go camping and huddle up in the tent together all night*
> *to put on your favorite music and sing and dance with you*
> *to plant our garden together and watch it grow*

*to scoop you up in my arms and tell you how very
much I love you every day every minute of every day*

TO PAUL, JUNE 6, 1990

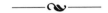

*You know something is wrong. I disappeared on you again
this morning, and you know I am worried. I can feel you put
up your walls so you don't get hurt again.*

*Oh, my sweet Paul. I want to be here for you every step of
the way . . . I want your happiness. I want you to feel safe and
secure and trust that I will always be here for you.*

Instead there is this uncertainty.

TO PAUL, SEPTEMBER 6, 1990

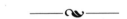

*I am wondering how all this will affect you. Will you come
not to trust life? Will this give you a greater resilience to overcome life's difficulties? . . .*

*I want life to be so good for you. I am so sorry to hand you
this. I only hope that something good will come of it for you.*

TO PAUL, FEBRUARY 28, 1991

*I have been writing most of this to the little Paul I know
and love, but I need to write a bit to the Paul who will read this
someday as a man.*

*So many times this year I have not known whether I
would live to see your second birthday. I have wanted to give
you security and a world you could trust. I have wanted you
never to feel abandoned. And I have been taken from you time
and time again.*

TO PAUL, MARCH 22, 1991

Is this the moral of *Sleeping Beauty*—no matter how much we try to protect our children, it's never really in our control? At some point we have to trust in the good fairies to hold them, even through the bad spells.

The possibility that I might die and leave Paul forever was just about more than I could stand.

———— ❧ ————

I can't tolerate the thought of what my dying would do to Paul. What does it mean to him that Mommy is gone? I can't bear for him to know that pain. Will he wonder what he did wrong? Would he think I didn't love him, that I didn't care? Would he cut himself off from his ability to love, to trust? I can't bear the thought of him being so damaged.

APRIL 12, 1991

———— ❧ ————

I need to be here for him. I want to be here for him.

Every day that I live, I think, that's one more day I've been able to give him.

I can't stand the thought of you wanting and needing your mama, and me not being here for you. And that's not something you'll grow out of by the time you're eight or twelve or sixteen. It's always there. And I want to be here as long as I possibly can.

DECEMBER 6, 1993

But there was another issue, which sometimes seemed bigger. I never ever wanted to have an only child. I grew up with so much love and companionship from my brothers and sister, and that continued as I grew older. Although I was told at age twenty that I probably would not survive a pregnancy, I never ever wanted my child to be so alone. I'd heard testimony from many friends who had been "only children" or parents of "only children" that it really can be a wonderful way to grow up, and for some children that might be true, but not Paul. He is not a solitary child and doesn't like solitary pursuits. He is happiest in a crowd, definitely a tribal animal, a puppy looking for the rest of the pack. He needs people to play with, a companion in life. He needs to be a brother. He has so much love to share and such a generous spirit—and he is so alone. This is not what I would have chosen for him. Of course, I could not have more children, as we had planned. We had to exercise birth *control*, and the adoption agencies we contacted would not talk with us.

—————☙—————

I feel so cheated of my life, and I feel David and Paul are cheated thereby too. More than anything I want to have another child. I was cheated of it in my youth and am cheated of it again now. Paul would be such a wonderful brother. And I can see him craving it. He is so intrigued by babies. And he always wants to go visit other children. He needs another child in his life, in his family. . . . How I wish I could give this to all of us.

NOVEMBER 2, 1991

This continues today. Age and medication prevent me from having another child now, and still our family doesn't feel complete. Still the roadblocks to adoption arise. Still Paul asks almost daily for a brother or sister. This is not what I had envisioned for him, or for us.

My body was out of control, not just with what was going on inside, but also with what was happening on the outside. I wasn't particularly enamored by my body shape and appearance. Like almost every other woman I know, I found fault with it in several places. But I had always been proud of my flat stomach. Pregnancy was worth the risk of losing it, but to my delight, it had come right back after Paul was born. Well, pride goeth before the fall. Now, it wasn't actually that my stomach wasn't flat. That would have been hard to tell because it had a large protruding box in it. The box was big and uncomfortable. Paul sometimes klonked his head on it. It even dictated my choice of clothes. It was hard to find anything to wear that would fit around it. Before the defibrillator was implanted, I'd always preferred to be tucked in and belted; afterwards I wore elastic waists and loose overshirts. I never felt like I could move right with this box in me. I had lost my grace. Even today, with the box removed, my stomach is out of my control. Though the box came out—and what a relief that was—the wires remained. I still have wires at my waist and a chunk of scar tissue in my stomach where the defibrillator was.

And the prednisone puffed my stomach up. As it did my face. In the first several months, my face was two to three times its normal size. This was hard. It was hard at first because I looked so fat, and I really had an encounter with fat prejudice in myself and others. For a long time, I was ashamed to be out in public. I didn't even like looking in a mirror. But what was harder than the vanity was the fact that no one knew me. People I had known for years passed me in the grocery store or in the halls of the university where I taught without acknowledgment. Many times I was carrying on a conversation with someone and realized that they didn't have a clue who I was; I'd have to introduce myself to someone I had known for over ten years. I suppose I could have had fun with this, but instead, not being known, not being recognized, just hurt. I didn't even recognize myself in the mirror. I missed my face. I missed me.

Then there was the hair. If my hair was any indication of what the medication was doing to the rest of my body—well, it was worrisome to say the least. The procainimide I was on to regulate my heart rhythm turned my brownish hair blond. This was okay. I'd been blond in my youth, and eventually I learned to like the color. But for a long time I was a punkish two-toned. Then just as I got used to being a blond, I had the transplant, stopped taking the procainimide, and started taking prednisone, which turned my hair black and white. Not only that, it made the straight crooked. My once straight hair was now quite wavy. And what had been thick hair before now got thicker. In addition, I was growing hair everywhere else on my body—my arms, my legs, my face, my stomach. My hair was out of control. Like my face, it was no longer mine. Perhaps it never had been.

Scars. The first scars on my hands from cut-downs for IVs when I was twenty were hard on my young body-conscious ego. Like my stomach, I'd fancied my hands one of my better features. The scars on them seemed to be big and purple for years. The next batch of scars on my chest and stomach weren't so bad. They were covered up most of the time. The chest scar was fairly unnoticeable under my breast, and the defibrillator itself was so noticeable and disfiguring, what did a few scars matter? But after the transplant surgery I just had to laugh. They'd carved out a road map on my body. Interstates down the center of my chest, unimproved roads across my stomach, a campground triangle symbol up by my shoulder. Any hope of body beautiful was gone; that's when I let go and simply celebrated my body for its capacity to carry me through life and for its resilience to all this trauma. I am proud of my scars. (Will this come to haunt me too?) I hope people will see them. This body is to be praised for all it has endured, and my scars are a testimony to that.

The laundry, the car, Paul's growing fascination with television, the color of my hair—these were little things, though often big and consuming at the time. But there were larger issues to deal with: my health, my life.

That my particular ailment was with my heart rhythm is so symbolic to me of the whole issue of control. With other illnesses there might be a vague sense of deterioration, but with mine, every minute— fifty, sixty times a minute—I was aware of whether my heart was beating correctly or not. Was it keeping the beat? Like a conductor I would count out the rhythm with the baton of my mind, and when it became irregular try to bring it along, back into rhythm. I have to laugh at myself now. On some level, I really thought if I focused on it hard enough, I could make it not skip that next beat. It was just a matter of concentration. I was heartened by the thought that some yogis can control their heartbeats. I was sure I could too. All my efforts at visualizing my heart on a swing were just more efforts to control it. But what could be a better lesson to me about what was and what was not in my control than my irregular and uncontrollable heart? I slowly began to admit that my heart's rhythm was beyond my control.

I did try to control my health in other ways. I tried to control it through a series of "if only's." In some bizarre thought process, I thought if I could rehash the past enough, perhaps I could change the present. If only I hadn't had my wisdom teeth out (which may have caused the initial damage to my heart). If only I'd taken steps to lower my blood pressure sooner. If only I'd taken heart meds sooner. If only... if only... if only... I spent hours going over these, trying to restore some kind of control in my mind. But rather than restoring control, it created regret, unhappiness, malcontent, and tension in my stomach. I was "if-onlying" myself to an ulcer, if not a heart attack.

I tried to control my health by controlling my treatment. First, I refused medication; then I demanded it. Ultimately I dictated which meds I would and wouldn't take. (I sensed my doctor was frustrated with me, though respectful of my wishes.) First I wanted the defibillator in; then I wanted it out. First I refused even to consider a transplant; then I clamored for one. Then I went round and round about whether or not the transplant was the right decision. First I had controlled through "if only's," now I was controlling through "what if's." What if the donor had AIDS? What if I got an infection? What if I rejected the heart? What if I went blind? Lame? You name it, I "what-iffed" it. I must have driven the doctors and nurses to distraction with my constant queries. I was trying to exercise some control by assuring myself this was the right decision, by seeking assurances where there were none to be had.

I never really made peace with the decision for the transplant. Up to the very last minute, I was questioning. One of the hardest letting go's in all of this was letting go of the known. We knew *this*; we knew this life with the defibrillator. It had its terrors, but they were familiar terrors. Going for the transplant was jumping into totally unknown territory. I could talk to people who'd had transplants, somehow thinking their lives would be mine. This was sometimes a comfort, sometimes not. A friend from high school had also needed a heart transplant, and he had died six weeks after surgery. Was his fate mine? One of my closest friends received a kidney transplant. He rejected at six weeks and needed a new kidney. With kidneys this is possible. One can go on dialysis until a new kidney is found. But with hearts . . . I tried to tell myself all the reasons why these wouldn't be my stories, but I didn't know. And that was the point. I didn't know. I had a vague road map at best. No road signs. This was a cliff, and I was expected to jump off it. Perhaps I had a rope, and perhaps I didn't. I wouldn't know until I jumped.

I wanted to know what to hope for. This involved magical thinking—that if I knew the right direction for my hope, I could hope this into being. I could wish it on a star or blow it on a birthday candle, and magically it would appear. After all, I'd wished for David, and he appeared; I'd wished for Paul, and he appeared. But now I didn't know what to wish for—to keep this old heart and heal it, or to let it go and hope that a new one would come soon.

This was the hardest letting go of all—letting go of my heart itself.

Last night I dreamed they called me for the transplant . . . I remember feeling relieved and ready. The time felt right. My mother was there . . .

Then I was suddenly gripped by the bizarre aspect of it all. I kept saying, "They're going to cut out my heart." It seemed like far too radical an idea, and I kept asking every person I met whether they thought it was a good idea.

It is a bizarre thought. They're going to cut my heart out! How can that possibly be a good thing to do?

DECEMBER 27, 1992

Cut my heart out! What an absurd proposition! How could I let go of this heart? Not only was it the central vital organ of my body, pumping lifeblood to all the others, but it was my friend, my beloved, the heart of all the loves and the heartaches and the trials and tribulations and joys of my life. We had been through so much together. How could I let them cut it out, cut it up, throw it away? This was my heart, that familiar pumping inside my chest. It was palpable, knowable. We had had many heart-to-heart talks, and in our heart-to-hearts she told me of her weariness, her fatigue. She had been steadfast. My God, she had endured so much shocking, surgery, disease, and heart-break. She was so tired. How could I let her go? How could I not? There comes a time when the most loving thing to do is to let go. Mother, Father, Mulford, June (my dear departed family, friend, and dog). Let them go, like the flowers in the fall, like the tears that fall from my face. Let them go; let them go. Their waters belong in Mombasa.

Perhaps this, this cutting out of my heart, was the most profound letting go. What an act of faith that was, to let them cut my heart out.

In my course of healing, my therapist urged me to do whatever I needed to let go. I was not able to let any healing take place because I was clinging so hard to life. I was fighting against death in a way that was creating more stress in my life. It was not healing.

So, finger by finger, I uncurled each one—each bit of unfinished business, each good-bye, each bit of resentment and regret—till I was ready. I wrote letters to people to whom I needed to say good-bye. Some were to those long gone from my life, and when I had written them I tore them up and scattered them like rose petals in the stream near my home. I wrote good-bye letters, somewhat disguised, to my brothers and sister. Perhaps they didn't know my true intent. David never liked the written word, so I spoke my heart to him as often as I could, though I did leave one good-bye letter for the time of my trans-plant. I wrote several letters to Paul: three for the transplant (which he never got—so much for my control!); a final good-bye letter; a letter to be opened when he turned thirteen; one for his wedding; and one for the birth of his first child; as well as the journal I kept, and con-tinue to keep, for him. Looking back through these journals, I can always tell when my rhythm felt critical. I would write one sentence only, the same sentence each time, "I love you always."

An envelope marked "In the event of my death . . ." sat on my desk. Included in its contents were my financial statements, the direc-tions as to the disposition of my things, and instructions for my me-morial service. Again I have to laugh at myself and my trying to con-trol even this from beyond my death. Will. We write wills to assure that our willfulness lives on. As I wrote directions about where I wanted my ashes scattered, I simply smiled at myself and ended up writing "put them wherever you would most want them to be. . . . Just be sure to put them with Juniper's (my soulmate/dog/companion)." I just couldn't let go all the way.

All this preparation for my death did help. I felt a definite sense of relief when I had finished.

In some ways, this preparation continued on a daily basis, in that I never put off anything anymore. I didn't know when I'd have another chance to say, or do, anything. I first learned this lesson years earlier when, at age twenty-one, I suffered my first cardiac arrest. I had a brief memory of lapsing into unconsciousness just before the arrest, so when I woke up in the emergency room, I knew something was terribly, terribly wrong. I could hardly breathe. I had vomited during my first husband's lifesaving efforts at CPR and had aspirated the vomit. My father had come to be with me in the emergency room. I sensed I might die at any time and I wanted him to know that I loved him, so I kept repeating, "I love you, Dad. I love you, Dad. I love you, Dad." I wanted to be sure that he heard me, that he knew. I have never put off telling someone I love them ever since. I learned to say the things I need to say. Often we don't say certain things, we keep silent out of a need to control. To be open is to be open to vulnerabilities, to visibilities. But as Audre Lorde said, they are "the visibilities without which we cannot truly live." We have a deep need to be visible, to be known— both to make a testimony of our lives and to have someone bear witness to that testimony.

As I came to grips with my illness and possible early death, I learned all these things, and I acted on them. Yet, despite all my best efforts at letting go, my heart still beat wildly. And I still had the sense of being totally out of control. I had recurring dreams of my car going out of control, driving over cliffs, off embankments, crashing into other cars. My car was my life. It had a will of its own.

As did my letting go. My most profound letting go's were effortless. And profoundly peaceful. I first felt this profound peace of deep letting go with that first cardiac arrest when I was twenty-one. In the hours preceding the arrest, my heart had been particularly bad. I sent my husband for my medication, and in the brief span of time between the moment he left to get my pills and the moment he returned to find my heartbeat and breathing stopped, I let go of life. In that letting go, I felt the deep peace, the profound embrace of the universe. I felt held in the palm of God's hand, as only a baby can be held.

I felt that deep peace one other time, when the stitch on the aorta slipped after my transplant surgery and I was bleeding to death. Though I remember little of the days immediately after my transplant surgery, this brief moment remains one of the most vivid memories of my life. This was the edge—between life and death. Not the final hours, but the final minutes. I knew that if nothing intervened, in a matter of minutes, perhaps seconds, I would die. This was it. I struggled with this for but a moment, willing myself to go on, and then I let go. Let go into the most gracious loving hands. This was God's will, God's way, the benevolent universe, deep loving peace. This was letting go. No fear here. This is goodness. This is greatness. The largeness of love.

"Tell Paul I love him," I said one last time. They assured me I could tell him myself. I still needed to say good-bye. Was it one last effort at control? Or was this one final letting go?

One final stick of the dam.

Let it go. Let it flow. Unbuild the dams, stick by stick, stone by stone if you must, but let the water flow. Therein lies the letting go.

Somewhere in all of this, I realized that letting go is not so much a leap of faith as a fall. And it isn't a fall into an abyss. It is a fall into a deep pool, with trust that the water will buoy you up. A fall into a deep pool of trust. It doesn't feel so much like God's will, as God's well. I don't often think of God as having a will, despite "thy will be done." It is too anthropocentric; it makes God too much a creation of human will. However, it makes things easier for us humans. God becomes our scapegoat, the one we can blame when things go wrong, and on whom we can lay a culpability that is rightly our own. When we will a willful God, it renders too much possibility of evil and judgment in the world. Perhaps God is trust itself—a deep-flowing bottomless stream. Perhaps God doesn't know the direction either, and simply calls on us to ride the current in trust, open to the wisdom of the universe.

It seems to me that that's what prayer is about—trust, openness. I had been frustrated with not knowing what to hope for, not knowing what to pray for, till I realized that the point wasn't for me to tell God what to do, but rather for me to listen. If anything, prayer is a dialogue, a call and response. Letting go is listening to the response. The trust is in heeding the wisdom. I trust that that wisdom is always out there, or more appropriately, in here.

The sin of pride lies in the arrogance of the belief that one's reason or one's will or one's fears know better than that greater wisdom. My life has not turned out as I planned, nor has my child's. There are days I rail against it, and when I do, it's because I think I know better than the universe. Yet, it seems so many of the miracles and blessings of life are things we didn't plan on. The best words I write are ones that just come, rather than the ones I agonize over. I think of the miracle of Paul, and that if I'd the children I'd planned, I wouldn't have him. Would I really have wanted it any different? I think of the blessings of family and friends and faith and perhaps a bit of wisdom that I have gained through my ordeal, and wonder, could I have planned for this?

Letting go is a matter of being open to the wisdom—letting go, taking out dams, flowing like a river. That is not to say it is a matter of following whims. There is a difference between whimsy and wisdom, between a settled and a surface desire, between currents and waves. It is not even necessarily a matter of doing whatever your heart tells you. There seems to be a place where the paths of heart wisdom and head wisdom cross. There is will and there is thoughtfulness—a confluence of the streams.

There are the days I listen, and the days I don't. I know the difference. The days that I don't, I put up roadblocks of directives and detours and haste. I don't want to take the turn it tells me. Those are clamoring, clanking, clinging days. The days I listen, I am open and everything flows. I think of an old friend who lives thousands of miles away; she calls from her daughter's house a mile down the road to say she wants to come visit. I pull a book from the shelf; it is just what I need to read. I feel a direction in my life, and get something in the mail showing me how to follow up on it. These are days of openness—joyful, jubilant, flowing free.

This lesson of trust and of openness came home strongly to me in the last weeks before the transplant.

——— ∞ ———

I feel that I am about to stop this whole process—and then I get flashes of what having a good heart would mean—everyday things like walking to my friends' houses and twirling around the living room with Paul. What a wonderful feeling to dive into the water and swim with abandon, frolicking in the waves. To skate hard and fast. To teach with passion. To climb to the top of a high hill. To dance. To live in trust of the rhythms of my heart.

If the "dry run" has taught me anything, it is that I must go into that operating room with full confidence and trust—with faith and with hope—with clarity and with an openness to the healing powers of the universe. I must focus on the faith rather than the fear, and let myself be held by the love and spirit of all the loved ones who surround me.

JANUARY 2, 1994

To focus on the faith, rather than the fear. To swim this river of my life with abandon. To be held in this deep pool by love. To live in trust of the rhythms of my heart.

Humility

———— ❧ ————

I have no doubt that it has been the generous prayers of so many that have kept me alive and so well for this long. Something far beyond me is sustaining me through all this. The power and the generosity and the love overwhelm me at times . . . How could I not but be humbled . . .

OCTOBER 20, 1992

In the years following being stricken with heart disease in my twenties, I carried a secret pride that I, I had cured the sickness in my heart. I had gone from being deathly ill to climbing mountains in Scotland. I had made my body well and strong. I had done this. I had done something right. I had believed enough. I had trusted enough. I had been pure enough. "Blessed are the pure in heart." My self-healing was a testimony to my righteousness on some spiritual plane. Maybe somewhere I shared the glory with a greater power than my own, but mostly I thought a lot of myself.

It was quite a blow to my pride to realize I wasn't cured, but far from being humbled by this realization, I picked up that ball of arrogance and ran with it again. If my heart were sick again, then I had done something to make it that way. And if I had made it sick, then I could make it well again. All of my initial attempts at self-healing were

61

exercises in arrogance. I have to laugh now at the arrogance of my "my will be done" attitude.

You'd think three cardiac arrests would have knocked the arrogance out of me, but in a way they did the opposite. I have often made the joke that because I've come back from the dead so many times, I'll be very surprised when I really do die. In the midst of all my fears of mortality, I also had a feeling of being immortal. People kept saying I must be alive for a reason. I kept looking for some grand purpose to my life. I must be very special indeed. I'd been practically resurrected. Certainly the transplant has been like a resurrection. But the point of resurrection is not to say, "I am Lord," but simply to have a chance to live better, more humbly.

Humble. Humus. We're all compost. My body will die someday—yes, I am in touch with that bit of reality—and become a part of the earth. Some people are put off by the thought of cremation or of being thrown into the earth without a coffin. I've always been bothered by the thought of being put in a box and being unable to breathe. Let my ashes be mixed with the earth and the water. Let me become as I have always been—humus—as much made of the earth as every other creature, leaf, and grain of sand.

Humus—the rich organic part of the soil. The life-giving part without which seeds won't sprout, flowers won't bloom, trees won't bear fruit, nothing will grow.

Dirt. It has such a bad name. When we treat people "like dirt," we treat them with contempt. Dirt. The giver of all life. We are all made of dirt. The food that sustains us grows only in the dirt—and the dirt is made of the stuff of stars. We are all made of stars.

Looking at the stars has always been an experience of both glory and humility for me. When I survey this glorious creation, I think that I must be very special indeed to be a part of this, and I am at the same time so humbled by my smallness in all of the vastness.

This, it seems, is the experience of humility. It is not about being treated like dirt. It is recognizing oneself as part of the dirt, as a particle of dirt like all the others, and knowing that dirt is the very substance of life. Both exceedingly special, and no more special than all the other particles.

It is the way a mother loves her children. I always felt I was precious to my mother, and though I sometimes wanted to be most precious, I never felt that I was more precious to her than the rest. She somehow loved us all equally. I was always amazed that she could do that. She would go to extraordinary lengths for each of us individually. I felt very special, yet no more so than my brothers and sister.

So has this been the lesson of my illness. Not the shame of wrongdoing, of being cast out, of being a leper, an untouchable; nor an arrogance of wellness in thinking myself above this. I needed to learn to walk a middle ground—to know that all are exceedingly special, and none more special than the rest.

When I first got sick in my twenties, I felt ashamed of my condition. I was so different from everyone else my age. I didn't want anyone to know there was anything "wrong" with me. I closeted my illness. Later that shame turned to self-blame in my self-accusations of sin and wrongdoing.

But I have known the other side too. Going to rehabilitation in my thirties always brought out my arrogance. What was I doing here with the old and infirm, I queried. I was young. I was strong. I didn't belong here. My arrogance continued after the transplant. I thought I was special. I was strong and well now. I didn't need to be in this clinic. I was cured, and didn't need to be here with all these sick people. I remember feeling that arrogance quite vividly on a day I had come to the clinic to get yet another biopsy. I thought little of the biopsy itself because, of course, *I* wouldn't reject. The next day they called to tell me I was rejecting.

Death—the great equalizer.

I was not special, meaning I was not above this. I was not above harm. I was as capable of being struck with plague as any other. There was no great shield of protection around me. I was no better than any of these hundreds of other hurt and dying people.

Today, as I walk around the University Hospitals and Clinic, I am struck by the way in which illness touches us all—the bald-headed children, the infants yellowed by jaundice, the old with gnarled bones, as well as those of us in our so-called prime with seeming vigor rendered not so vigorous. I see the many hues of black and brown, dark and pale. I hear the tongues of many nations—Hmong, Chinese, English, Spanish, Czech. We are all there assembled. None is spared. All are touched. Even saints sicken and die. No one is spared by age, by race, by religion, by sex, by all those things that separate us. We all take our turn in line.

Though not spared the vicissitudes of illness and death, one group is markedly absent from the transplant line—those unable to pay for their treatment. While efforts are made to secure funding, those who cannot pay on their own or through insurance cannot join the line, and this distinction will always bother me.

Each of us a particle of dirt. Each of us a star. For all of us who assemble in this place, extravagant measures are undertaken for the sustaining of our lives. This effort to keep me alive has been most humbling. When I think of the lengths to which strangers have gone to keep me alive; when I think of the expense—the hundreds of thousands of dollars; when I think of all the effort and energy and intelligence and tenacity and training; when I think of the many resources—each syringe, each X ray, each pill, each IV solution; when I think of all the medical personnel—the paramedics, the nurses, the doctors, the X-ray technicians, the lab technicians, the pharmacists, the nutritionists, the many who prepare my meals and clean up my bedpans, the EP team, the transplant team, the CCU teams—when I think of all this, I cannot help but wonder how one life could be worth all of this. You would think I were High Queen.

And most of these amazing efforts occurred before the transplant itself. The first time I heard a nurse from LifeSource describe the coordination of efforts involved in procuring, transporting, and implanting a transplanted organ, I was in total awe. Awe that this is done for so many; awe that this had been done for me.

Computerized systems match donor to recipient. Transplant teams travel, sometimes hundreds of miles, to remove the organs and transport them to their various recipients, who may themselves be traveling by air or land ambulance, unless already hospitalized. The nurses and surgeons are called from their rounds or their son's recital or their daughter's soccer game or their beds. The timing, the planning, the transportation, the expense, the effort—comparable to that of a huge wedding or gala that takes months or years to prepare—are all coordinated in a few hours time. All of this so that one, two, maybe six more people will have a chance for restored health and life. All of this done for me—and not just once, but twice, and all this before the transplant even takes place. How could I or anyone be this important?

But all of this, all the coordination and effort, seems but little when I think of the fact that my life is sustained through the life of another, that someone else's heart beats inside my body. All the efforts of so many people make this possible, but the time comes when the surgeons have done all they can, and they simply must wait for the heart to beat on its own.

We all have known something of this. All of us began this life journey sustained by the heart and lifeblood of our mothers. All that mothers endure to bring forth new life is equally humbling. Nothing I know of is so directly akin to the original holding in the womb as this, another's heart giving me life. Right after the transplant I imaged my holding this heart as if she were a child in my womb, for that is the one time nature allows a stranger inside our bodies without rejecting it. Now I see the relationship is really the other way around, or perhaps it is a mutual holding.

Being sustained through another's heart cannot but be humbling. What could more directly contradict the idea of a self-sufficient, independent existence than this? No longer can I lapse into the mindless arrogance of thinking anything entirely *my* doing. I am only because *we* are: "We are, therefore I am."

We all sustain each other. We are not alone, self-sufficient.

Not long ago, one of my students asked if I believed in God. I responded that I did, though my conception of God was probably quite different from hers. I said something to the effect that I could not have been through all that I had, and not believe in a power beyond my own.

Another of my students tried to talk me out of my belief, arguing that it could have been the strength of my own human will that helped me to overcome my adversity. I understand what he meant. Certainly I credit my will to live as essential in keeping me alive during my greatest trials. I never quietly slipped away without a fight, but I actually hadn't had those times of crisis in mind. I'd been talking about a power that sustained me over the long haul. I was talking about the cradle of arms in which I was carried when my heart was too weary and the road too long.

During my waiting time, my minister had given me a journal on lamentations of the heart to help me with the feeling she imagined I must have of "God, why hast thou forsaken me?" But the truth was, I never felt forsaken. Whenever I asked for strength to endure one more hour or one more day—at those points when I felt I could not go another step—I was carried. I was carried by the prayers and energies of many. I have known the feeling of being held by many, many hands and hearts, all woven in a web of comforting, loving, peaceful prayer. I have felt the energy encircling, enfolding, holding me up and through. I would pray simply for strength—and it was always offered. It was as if I handed my burdens over. I felt a strength beyond my own. Beyond my own will. Far from being a matter of my own will, I experienced this as something quite radically other than my own will, a "meta" will.

I am not here on my own power. I have been held through this. I have been carried. It is a palpable power.

To recognize and to honor a power beyond one's own seems the essence of humility. This acknowledgment carries with it that same quality of the dirt and the stars and mother love—to be at once so small among the greatness and so precious. To be small but not diminished; to be honored but not above any other.

The awareness of another's heart beating in my body is a continual exercise in humility. Every day I am called upon to recognize the limits of my individual existence, and the expansiveness of that existence in the interconnections with all of creation. I am so very aware of the smallness of my part in all of this, and I am so honored to be alive.

Mindfulness

———❧———

It is hard to be alone in the stillness and dreariness of this day. Every extra heartbeat beats so loudly. I want to turn down the volume on my awareness.

NOVEMBER 27, 1990

I n the months and years following my cardiac arrest, my heart was on my mind. It was not so at first. I had lived with cardiac dysrhythmia for all of my adult life. This chapter of my life was to be no different and I paid my heart little mind. However, the episode of incessant shocking, shortly after my defibrillator operation in 1990, zapped me to attention. Following that, my heart became like a Buddhist temple bell, calling my mind back from wherever it was to focus on the present moment of my heart. I began to count beats. One skipped beat was a warning, which left unheeded might lead to my being shocked—a subtle reminder, a bit unnerving, but livable. Five skips a minute and I began to grow tense. Beyond that, my sense of safety quickly eroded, and in those times when the PVCs would come every other beat or in couplets or triplets or more I would be off again to the emergency room. From time to time, I would lapse into mindless complacency; then like a child pulling at her mother's hem, my heart would tug and pull at my mind. If all else failed, thirty joules of electricity would quickly jolt me back to attention.

With each bout of severe dysrhythmia, with every tachycardia, with each shocking episode, my mind became more focused on my heart. I would try to carry on a conversation or pay attention to my child, but my heart tugged and pulled me away. You could post a sign on my mind that read "occupied." My mind was full—full of my heart. And it was full of anxiety and fear, which made my heart more irritable, which made me more anxious, which made my heart more irritable. Round and round we went. I needed to find a way through this.

When first diagnosed with heart failure shortly after Paul was born, I began meditating regularly to lower my blood pressure and bring about healing. With my mind focused on the sensations in my nose, head, and chest, I would breathe in, in, in, in, in, and out, out, out, out—all the way out until my breath came rushing back in—cleansing my body of negative energy, breathing in healing energy, feeling the deep calm settle in around me. I often found it hard to leave that place of quiet stillness. After awhile, I would turn my attention to my hands. By directing the flow of my blood, I could warm them, thereby dilating my blood vessels and taking the pressure off my heart.

I also used visualization to heal the scarred ventricle, reduce the size of my heart, and heal my mitral valve. Deep into a meditation, I would imagine my heart small and well and whole. I truly believed in my capacity to heal myself. (And while I was unable to heal my heart completely, my valve actually did heal, much to the astonishment of my doctors.)

Following my cardiac arrest and the operation to implant the defibrillator, I continued to practice meditation, but with a different purpose. I no longer believed I could quickly and easily heal the massive damage to my heart muscle simply by visualizing it so. I was struck by something Deepak Chopra had written about the deep-seatedness of chronic illness. It had taken twenty years for my heart to become so damaged; I could not expect it to be healed overnight. I did meditate to heal the damaged tissues of my heart, but my primary goal was to regulate my heart rhythm. I visualized myself on a swing, swinging back and forth in regular rhythm, and hoped that the rhythm of my heart would follow the rhythm of my mind. I also meditated to decrease my overall anxiety, to bring a backdrop of peacefulness and serenity into my life. This worked to a point. But as my heart steadily worsened, and with the memories of the shocking ever present, the point came when focusing on my breathing became impossible. In the stillness, my heart would seem to beat even louder. I would try to concentrate on my breathing, but my focus would inevitably shift to the beat of my heart. Beat, beatbeat, beat, beatbeatbeat—each beat shook my body. Every irregular beat pounded its dysrhythmic thump on my chest. It was a drum, beating wildly, erratically, and like a drum beating ever faster, louder, wilder, it both captivated and frightened me.

When my nephew John was a baby, he often awoke in the middle of the night. My sister would rock him, and the steady rhythm of the rocking and the familiar beat of her heart soon soothed him back to sleep. On a night she left him in my care, he awoke as usual, but the rocking did no good. As I held him close to my quite irregular heart, he screamed all the louder, so terrified he was of this wildness. He sensed the danger. So too now, when I held myself to my heart, I became frightened by its wildness, its erratic behavior. This was not soothing to me. I longed for the steady lubdub of my mother's heart, of my own heart. Instead, I knew only fear.

Obviously, meditation was not having its intended effect. Instead, it only intensified my fears. Meditation as I had practiced it needed to cease.

Nevertheless, I still needed to find a way through the fear, a way to calm myself. In my meditative practice, shifting the focus from my breathing to my hands took the pressure off my heart. So now, shifting my focus to my hands, to the work of my hands, took the pressure off my mind. My hands guided me through the fear.

My hands began cleaning . . . oh so slowly . . . washing every inch of counter, rinsing each dirty dish, putting away toys, hanging sheets and shirts and pillowcases.

Each task led to the next. And here, in the daily round of ordinary tasks, done slowly, with all of my attention focused on the doing of my hands, being here now, I found my peace.

My father-in-law had wanted to help us out by hiring someone to clean the house for us, but I refused his gift. Perhaps I instinctively knew the therapeutic value of these daily tasks of housecleaning, but I also felt they held spiritual value for me. It was important to me to stay in touch, literally, with the "lowly" tasks of life. In Colossians 3:12, Paul calls on the Colossians to put on a new nature—compassion, kindness, meekness, patience, and "lowliness." Lowliness. A willingness to be low. To do the lowly work. The necessary work. The tedious work. The daily work of keeping up with the growth and the decay and the dirt. The manual labor—the work of hands. The ancient Greeks considered this to be the work of slaves and of women, those unfit for the higher freedoms of the soul. Yet, this lowly work is soul work.

Lowliness. Staying low. Good advice when caught in a thunderstorm. Staying low to the ground keeps us from being shocked. In this thunderstorm of my life, staying low helped to ground me from shocks, quite literally, but it also helped to ground my being. Staying low, doing the lowly work, helps keep us spiritually grounded from the jolts and shocks of life. Perhaps this was the truth Gandhi knew in requiring everyone in his ashram to have their turn at doing the work of the "untouchable." Perhaps this spiritual grounding has something to do with humility, of not thinking oneself to be above any task. Perhaps it has something to do with not putting oneself above anyone else. Perhaps it has to do with not denying any of God's gifts. But for me, the spiritual gift was not so much in the task itself, but in the way I went about doing it—slowly, attentively, reverently—as if it were the only task that needed doing. It was this mindful attention to the task that brought the healing quality, the holy quality. Healing, wholeness, holiness. They are all present in the daily tasks that call for our attention.

For much of my life, I thought of spirituality as being somewhere "out there": transcendent. It is the spirit after all. One can't see it or taste it or hear it or touch it. But the more I live, the more I see it as being connected with the way I walk and talk and go about my daily tasks. The way I hug my child, wash dishes, and cut carrots has as much to do with spirituality as time spent in church or time spent in prayer. They embody the spirit.

My hands guided me elsewhere. My hands began to knit, and in the slow repetitive circular motion, the rough of the yarn against the smooth of the needle, the in and round and off, in and round and off, these hands showed me the way through my fears. When my heart began one of its irregular moods, I would pick up my knitting and let the slow patterned movement of my hands and the steady tension of the yarn draw out the tension in my mind and heart.

My hands led me to my garden. I longed for hard work that made my skin sweat and my muscles sore and my body good and tired, but took to the safer, less demanding task of weeding. I welcome weeds in my garden simply so I can pull them out—not the tough weeds with the deep tap roots, but the small and shallow ones that resist only slightly, and with a gentle tug relinquish their hold on the ground. Slowly, repetitively, meditatively, pull and release . . .

Pull and release, so did my hands tug on the strings of my harp. The sound board of the harp reverberated next to my heart, and somehow I think it did it good, but what drew me to the harp was the feel of it in my hands. There is something akin to the tension of the yarn and the tug and pull of the weed in the plucking of the harp string. Some resistance, some release. More than that, I found serenity in the configuration of my fingers over the strings, the movement of my fingers from one string to the next. As they moved across the strings, my hands brought me to a peaceful place.

What is it about hands? There is such power in them. The power to heal and the power to kill; the power to comfort and to crush, to create and destroy. Hands hold, hands let go, hands tell stories, hold babies, wrap presents, play pianos, bake cakes, wash socks, touch tenderly, hit hard, throw baseballs, plant seeds, make gifts.

The things that we make by hand hold a special almost spiritual quality. They are gifts from the heart. Christmas doesn't seem like Christmas when I don't make something by hand. It is the making by hand that invokes the spirit of the season. Handmade presents are treasures for both the giver and the recipient. In those years that I

soothed my soul with knitting, more than the motion of it was soothing, for I also knew I was making gifts for Paul, something of me and
of mine he could carry into his future, pass on to his children, even if
I weren't there. He could still hold a bit of my spirit in holding what
had been made by my hands.

Through our hands, we touch the world, simultaneously giving to
it and receiving from it. We convey so much by our touch: tenderness,
anger, indifference, lethargy, gentleness, comfort, despair. The sting of
a slap is more than the physical pain, being as well the hurt and hate it
carries with it, the palpable sensation of scorn. The comfort of a caress
is more than its physical softness; the comfort is the care and concern
it conveys.

Hands connect us to the world and to each other. We say we'll be
in touch. To be out of touch is to be unconnected, not communicat-
ing with each other. To be out of touch, to lose hold, is to lose our grip
on reality. Hands connect us to the real world. Not to have hands is
crazymaking.

I am reminded of the story of the handless maiden recounted by
Clarissa Pinkola Estes. In the story, a miller who had fallen on hard
times unknowingly bargains away his daughter to the Devil in ex-
change for untold riches. But when the time comes for the Devil to
come for her, the purity of her hands is so great that he is repelled. The
Devil orders the father to chop off her hands, which he does with great
reluctance. Still, the stumps of the daughter's arms are so pure, that
again the Devil is repelled and disappears. The daughter takes on the
life of a beggar, and spends years wandering through the forest. There
she meets and marries a king. The king leaves to wage war in a far-off
land, but in his absence, the young queen bears a child. A message is
sent to the king, but the Devil intervenes and sends a message back to
the king's mother to kill the queen and the child. Instead, the king's
mother sends the queen and her babe into the forest, where she again
wanders, but as she cares for her child, her hands grow back. Years
later she is rejoined by the king, who has also been wandering in the
forest searching for her.

We are told a story of the power of hands. The daughter's hands must be cut off because they are so powerful they repel even the magic of the Devil. But without her hands, the daughter is left wandering through the forests of life. She is out of touch, with her family, with her husband, with her soul.

In a particularly striking version of this story, as the queen bends over a well to draw water, the baby falls into the well. The queen, helpless without her hands, begins to scream.

> *A spirit appears and asks why she does not rescue her child. "Because I have no hands!" she cries. "Try," says the spirit, and as the maiden puts her arms in the water, reaching toward her child, her hands regenerate then and there, and the child is saved.*
>
> CLARISSA PINKOLA ESTES, *Women Who Run with the Wolves*

Estes goes on to talk about how the child represents the childself, the soulself. In reaching out to the child, the queen reaches out to her soul, and her hands grow back. Hands are vehicles to the soul.

In some ways, this was my story. My father didn't sell me to the Devil, and my hands weren't chopped off—though in my days of self-blaming, I could have imagined a vengeful Heavenly Father doing so—but I was disconnected, out of touch with my spiritual center, my days and nights spent wandering in fear-filled forests. My hands instinctively reached out and brought my childself, my soulself, to a restorative and peaceful place.

My hands were not alone in this. My feet led me to places I needed to go as well. Before my arrest, I walked at a brisk pace. I remember fairly racing my long-legged Ph.D. advisor, Mulford Sibley, over the Washington Avenue Bridge, and how we laughed as we discovered that each of us was trying to keep up with the other. In London, the group of students I was with found that the only way to keep peace among us was to divide up by pace. I went with the fastest walkers, and we traversed all of London and more in a day. My sister-in-law and I found ourselves to be good traveling companions simply because we were both "good walkers." And just hours before my arrest, I was walking briskly up and down hills with my baby boy in a pack on my back. How I loved the feeling of a good brisk walk, my body full of energy and bounce and enthusiasm.

Now this was gone. To walk fast was to risk raising my heart rate to a dangerously high level. I had to march, as it were, to a different and slower drummer. My brisk pace slowed to a stroll. My walks became rambles. Where I once knew the strength and vigor of a good tromp, I now knew the calm of slow steady walking, feeling the rhythm of my body in a new way, feeling the earth push back against my step, watching the sky, listening to birds. There was a peacefulness in this slower pace.

Late in my pretransplant saga, doctors implanted a new defibrillator in me. It included a pacing device, which would electronically pace my heart back to a slower rhythm, rather than shock me, which seemed to cause my heart to speed up. A pacing device was exactly what I needed, though not necessarily an electronic one. It seemed that my bodymind had found its own pacing device in the slow pace of my hands as I cleaned and knitted and weeded and in the slow pace of my feet in their rambles. I found as well the slower pace of a reduced load at work. Given smaller classes and fewer committee assignments, I had a less busy work life. I dropped most of my extracurricular involvements. My music had gone with my first cardiac arrest. My political crusades went with the second. Exercise classes and country dances were a thing of the past. And since I couldn't walk up and down the hills, even canvassing the neighborhood for the heart fund had to go. My only outside commitment was playing the piano for the children's choir at church, the one delight I couldn't part with. As the pace of my life changed, I found that it allowed for a serenity and an awareness that the speed and busyness of my full-time life had not. No longer would I respond to "How are you?" with the answer I had so often given in the past—"busy," (or "*too* busy"). I was glad for my slower pace. I was less irritable, more peaceful.

What I didn't know at the time was that I was intuitively practicing "mindfulness," the Buddhist practice of approaching each task with a deliberateness—a presence of mind—an engagement of the mind completely on the present. To be mindful is to be fully attentive to someone or to the task at hand.

I discovered the works of Thich Nhat Hanh—*The Miracle of Mindfulness, Being Peace, Touching Peace.* In these he gives exercises in mindfulness—mindfulness while making tea, while cleaning the house, while taking a bath, while washing the dishes:

> *Wash the dishes relaxingly, as though each bowl is an object of contemplation. Consider each bowl as sacred.*
> *Follow your breath to prevent your mind from straying.*
> *Do not try to hurry to get the job over with. Consider washing the dishes the most important thing in life.*
>
> THICH NHAT HANH, *The Miracle of Mindfulness*

Consider washing dishes the most important thing in life. How often do we do that? How often do we ever consider what we are doing to be the most important thing in life? Yet, the message of mindfulness is that everything we do is the most important thing. Everything is deserving of our full attention.

Every moment is our life. All that we do is our life. It is in honor and respect of that life, of our creation, that we approach it mindfully.

After discovering the works of Thich Nhat Hanh, I practiced the exercises in mindfulness in a more deliberate manner. I extended my mindfulness from cleaning and knitting to bathing and brushing my teeth and cutting vegetables. . . .

The shower was a particularly hard place for me. In the hospital, it seemed that the first test of strenuous activity was always taking a shower. If I could do that without trouble, then I could go home. At home, I always worried that raising my hands above my head, scrubbing my hair, would be too hard, that my heart would go too fast, that I would be shocked, and that with the water running no one would hear me yell for help. I began the practice of mindfulness in the shower—feeling the warmth and pressure of the water, listening to the "whoosh" as it came out of the showerhead, feeling each drop as it ran down my body, feeling the slipperiness of the soap. It did soothe my mind, when I could remain present to it.

Though I adopted mindfulness as a meditative exercise to overcome my anxieties and focus my mind, and it did help me to do this, I discovered it was a vehicle to so much more. Buddhists practice mindfulness not simply as a celebration of creation, but as a meditative vehicle through which to become and engage peace, serenity, compassion, loving kindness. I think of the times when I am most irritable, most likely to snap a response, become impatient. It is when my attention is divided—when I am trying to listen to both my husband and my son at the same time; when I need to be out the door and the phone is ringing; when a student needs to talk and I am trying to get material ready for class. It is the pulling in two or several directions at once, making me unable to give my attention to none, that makes me irritable. Mindfulness, attention to the task or the person at hand, brings me through, shows me the way to be at peace, to know compassion, to act in loving kindness.

But even more than this, mindfulness became a way of claiming my life.

> *If while washing dishes, we think only of the cup of tea that awaits us, thus hurrying to get the dishes out of the way as if they were a nuisance, then we are not "washing the dishes to wash the dishes."*
>
> *What's more, we are not alive during the time we are washing the dishes.*
>
> THICH NHAT HANH, *The Miracle of Mindfulness*

My life was threatening to be too short as it was. I did not want to squander those moments I did have by letting my mind wander away from the only life I had, the life I was living here and now. But I did that so often. I think of the many times driving down the highway that I have been startled to discover I was several miles down the road from my last awareness of where I was. I've played whole pieces on the piano with no awareness of playing them; read several pages of books with no awareness of the words.

How often are we fully attentive to the present moment? I tested this on my students one day. At random moments during class I rang a Buddhist meditation bell, and asked them to stop and tell me where they were. At any given time, only about a third of them were there in that classroom. The rest were on to their next class already, or back in yesterday's conversation, or in Minneapolis, or Cub Foods, or back in bed.

I think of the many times when I would be reading to Paul, finding I'd read the whole book (which I had undoubtedly read a hundred times before) without being aware of it. My mind would be going over a conversation I'd had that day or planning what I would do after he was asleep—and I would realize that I had just wasted my precious time with my son, for though I was there in body, I was not present to him. Mindfulness became a reminder to me of the preciousness of the present moment. It became a way in which I could claim my life from the grasping hands of fear and death.

To live mindfully is to live fully in the present moment. Even if my life were to be short, if I lived every moment in full awareness of the present moment then I would in a sense have more of it. And if we do not do this, then what is life but a dream, a phantom? I am reminded of my son, who all of his life has resisted sleep because there is so much living to do. Why should we not also refuse to spend our waking life asleep to the moment, when there is so much living to do?

The preciousness of life comes easily after a transplant. Life is new and sweet. Each moment is to be savored. With the mindfulness of a child (which so often seems like mindlessness to grown-ups), one can spend hours just looking at clouds. There is so much to delight in.

Yet, mindfulness is the lesson I am most likely to forget now that I have my new heart. I feel like I have to make up for "lost" time, and that I don't know how much time I'll have to do that. I am in such a hurry to do all the things I did not have a chance to do in all those years of disability, and to do them quickly before my reprieve is over. The pressure to be up and doing can be so strong. But then I remember the "lost" time, and know that it was not really lost. I got less done, but was that so important? Sometimes I wonder about our preoccupation with getting things done. Yes, there are the tasks imposed by necessity. But beyond that, we have choices to make, and it seems we often choose doing over being. Not that they are separate and apart from each other in any event. Philosopher Sam Keen writes, "From our being flows our doing." Who we are and how we are becomes what we do. The quality of our doing follows from the quality of our being. Of what value to the world is work done in haste and pressure? Does the stress created in such creation ultimately destroy—health, relationships, harmony—more than it creates? Why must we always be so busy? What is it that we aren't paying attention to, that we don't want to pay attention to? Why are we in such a hurry? We say it's because we don't want to waste time. But I know that in the rush of busyness I waste more time, because I am not able to be present to it. How little do we recognize the preciousness of time? We squander it. Our busyness keeps us from being fully present to the present moment. And we are irritable. We waste each other's lives. We do violence to ourselves and to each other. A more peaceful world requires a slower pace.

I'm back to work full time, with a full load and more, back to being involved with my church and school and community. My life is fast-paced, as is my walk, walking as I now do for a good aerobic workout. It is easy to let mindfulness slip away. Yet, the lesson of mindfulness has carried through in certain respects. My life has its busy moments, but more often I would describe it as full. I notice the slower pace I take now with my work. It "takes" more of my time, but it is taken in a new depth. It has a meditative quality I didn't know before. I'm not rushing it. I follow it where it leads me. It is more demanding than stressful, and it feels good.

My best days with Paul are the days we don't have to go anywhere, do anything. We set our own pace. We flow from baking cookies to playing Chutes and Ladders to dancing to being alone together.

I still find a peacefulness in cleaning (when I get to it).

And every once in awhile, I go for a ramble.

We walk all the time, but usually it is more like running.
When we walk like that,
we print anxiety and sorrow on the Earth.
We have to walk in a way that we only print
peace and serenity on Earth. . . .
When we are able to take one step peacefully, happily,
we are for the cause of peace and happiness
for the whole of humankind.

THICH NHAT HANH, *Being Peace*

Hope

———— ◈ ————

I have been going round and round all night about whether to go ahead with the transplant. I only know I felt relieved when my doctor said he thought I should go ahead with it. This morning the words that come to me are from the play The Diary of Anne Frank. *As the gestapo pull up to the building where the Franks have been hiding, Otto Frank says, "For two years we have been living in fear, now we can live in hope." Now we can live in hope.*

APRIL 29, 1992

On an afternoon in July of 1991, I walked out of the University of Minnesota Clinic in abject despair. "Go home and see how it goes next time," they said. See if I'm tortured next time. See if it kills me next time. There's no way out. I'm trapped. I climb the walls of my cell/soul entombed in my body. No way out. No way. No, no, no . . . I am blanketed with gloom. I stand there motionless, for there is no motion—no going forward, no going back. My life is at a standstill and I stand still there wondering what is the point of going on. If this horror is to be my life, and I will die of it sooner or later, then better that it be sooner and have it done with. On this bright sunny day in July with people laughing and busily going about their lives all around me, the world lost its color, and I lost all desire to live. On that day, I lost my last hope. They had denied me a transplant.

A transplant is a gift of life for those lucky enough to make it that far, but for those waiting for a transplant, it is a gift of hope. Hopefulness is the essential quality of those seeking a transplant. To have that hope denied was to plunge me into the colorless world of George Orwell's *1984*—a world of torture and control and joyless existence. "We are the dead." Yes, to live without hope was to exist as one already dead.

A few weeks later when they rethought their decision and okayed the transplant, the color came back to my world. My hope had been restored. For two years I had been living in fear—fear of being tortured by shocks, fear of losing my mental capacities, fear of dying and leaving my loved ones, fear of spending the rest of my life in fear—and that fear kept me in hiding from the world. Now I could live in hope. Oh, the fear came and went throughout that time of waiting. Indeed, I feared the very thing I hoped for. Yet, through all my questioning of the transplant decision, at bottom I chose it. Every time I imagined going forward in this life without it, I fell into my colorless world. I feared that gray world of no hope most of all. It was hope that made living with and through my fears possible. Without hope, I could not have gone on. This is the gift of hope—the ability to go on.

"We go on," writes songwriter Claudia Schmidt. Her music circles my heart with hope and encourages me to go on . . .

> . . . *canoe under hot sun,*
> *the upturned paddle guides liquid to our dry mouths,*
> *water within us, water surrounds us, a great mystery,*
> *our becoming dry at all . . . replenish,.*
> *all must be replenished,*
> *the water within and without, all that fills us,*
> *all that surrounds . . .*
> *the great whistling pines, the tenacious beaver,*
> *the ancient loon,*
> *the rush of the young eagle's wings*
> *as it dips low over our canoe . . .*

replenish the eyes bathed in this delicate solitude,
this trembling eternity called back in mid-sweep
only to be assessed by greed-parched eyes . . .
replenish each shriveled heart which has its moments
only at events set aside for its song,
but cannot fly for the connection between the rock
and the human body, the heron's wing
and the hope in our souls . . .
we go on, our paddles dance with the lake water
to the music in our throats . . .
we will grow dry again, perhaps leap into the water,
a small and symbolic celebration of a great and endless task
which, gracefully undertaken, might allow us all to go on,
and on, and on. . . .

CLAUDIA SCHMIDT, "Replenish"

Like Sisyphus and his rock, I had this great and endless task of life before me, and that rock seemed to keep tumbling down—one setback after another, one disappointment after another, one more day of dysrhythmia, one more day of waiting and wondering. Sometimes I wanted to lie down and let this shriveled heart rest, and each time hope replenished my shriveled heart and allowed me to go on and on. Hope carried me through the dark times. There were plenty of dark times, and without the hope of the transplant, I don't know that I could have gone on. During those times, I occasionally would literally envision my future with a new heart, and all that would mean. I would see myself hiking, running on the beach, dancing, being bravely out in the world, embracing life. But usually hope did not carry a specific image or thought. Rather, hope came as a feeling of strength, of being lifted up from the inside. When I thought I couldn't go on, hope would carry me. There is a fortitude in hope that carries us through adversity.

In Romans 5:3–4, Paul calls on us to rejoice in our sufferings: "Knowing that suffering produces endurance, and endurance produces character, and character produces hope." But I think Paul got some of this backwards. It is not suffering that produces endurance, and endurance that produces hope. Rather, it is hope that enables one to endure suffering.

In all of this, my most acute suffering came when I was being shocked. Hope for me then was the sirens' song. They sang of the hope that help was near, hope that the torture would soon end, hope that I would make it through again. That hope carried me through. I remember in particular that day in June when I was shocked after planting on my hillside. I was sitting on the couch, Nancy by my side, my heart beating faster and faster, fearful of being shocked again and then came that lovely sound of sirens. I could hang on now. Help was near. And then just as I was encouraged, so was I dismayed as the siren faded away. Hope was indeed lost. Finally, the sound grew closer once again and gave me enough hope to hang on a while longer. I cannot hear a siren now without being brought back to those days of fear. Sometimes tears come to my eyes. The sound brings back my fear, but also my hopes. Yes, we can make it now.

On a daily basis, my nights were the hardest. My rhythm was always worse with the fatigue of the day, and my anxiety seemed to grow with the dark. "Joy may come with the morning" (Psalm 30:5), but hope is what carries us through the night. As the words of the Welsh hymn remind me:

> *Though our hearts be wrapt in sorrow,*
> *From the hope of dawn we borrow*
> *Promise of a glad tomorrow,*
> *All through the night.*
>
> "All Through the Night"

Though my heart was wrapped in sorrow, the hope of the dawn carried me through each night, just as the hope of the dawn of a new life carried me through that dark night of my life.

Suffering without hope will not be long endured. Suffering without hope kills the spirit before it kills the body. Anne Frank lived those years in hiding with the great hopefulness of youth: "In spite of everything I still believe that people are really good at heart." I imagine it was her hopefulness in the human spirit that helped her to endure that time of hiding. Yet, it is said that in the last days of her life in the concentration camp, she had become despondent, without hope. I imagine she no longer believed in the essential goodness of people's hearts. She had no hope, and succumbed fairly quickly to disease. We cannot live long without hope.

The worst thing a doctor can tell a patient is that their case is hopeless. Without hope, the spirit dies, and then what does it matter of the body? Just as Steven Levine suggests that rather than ask, "Should I heal?" we ask, "Where does the healing lie?" so might we rather than ask, "Is there any hope?" ask, "Where does the hope lie?" Even for the terminally ill patient, hope can be found.

When I was training to volunteer for hospice, in a session on hope, we were posed the situation of a terminally ill patient and asked where does the hope lie. I thought of a woman I had known named Kay. She was younger than I at the time I knew her, probably nineteen or twenty. And she had terminal cancer. She had exhausted every hope—every hope for not physically dying, that is, but not her hope for living. On what turned out to be the last night of her life, her husband fulfilled her repeated request that they go swimming. He lowered her frail tiny body into the water and for a while she was free of the disease, free of the fear. She was alive. She lived out her hope. She lived well into her death. Can any of us hope for more?

Poet, playwright, and now president of the Czech Republic Vaclav Havel writes:

> *Hope is a state of the mind, not of the world. . . .*
> *Hope, in this deep and powerful sense,*
> *is not the same as joy that things are going well,*
> *or willingness to invest in enterprises that are obviously*
> *heading for . . . success,*
> *but rather an ability to work for something because*
> *it is good,*
> *not just because it stands a chance to succeed.*

VACLAV HAVEL, "The Politics of Hope"

While it may be nourished by success, or even by the good odds of succeeding, hope does not require the likelihood of success. Hopefulness is being able to look at a 95 percent failure rate and hope to be in the 5 percent. Hopefulness is knowing death is imminent and finding a way to live well in that knowledge.

For me, the question, "What if the transplant doesn't work?" nagged at the back of my mind. That possibility was pretty devastating to me. It contributed to much of my dilemma. But despite that real possibility, I went on. Despite all of its difficulties, despite the fact that I might die on the way to getting the transplant itself, or on the table, or a few weeks after, the transplant represented hope to me. As much as I could not live long without a new heart, neither could I live long without the hope of one. Every time I thought of abandoning the transplant, of living without that hope, I fell into despondency. The hope carried me through.

I imagine donor families might feel bad to learn that the person to whom they donated their loved ones' organs died soon after transplant. They might feel that they had given nothing at all. But it's not true. Even had I died on the table that night, I would have had the hope that carried me through as far as I had come. It had kept my spirit alive. A transplant is a gift of hope. From a medical standpoint, the value of the transplant hinges primarily on whether or not it succeeds in extending the life of the patient. From a spiritual standpoint, inasmuch as the transplant gives hope, it is already a success.

There is a story in Revelations about a portent of a woman who is in the throes of labor, when another portent appears in the sky, this time of a dragon. "And the dragon stood before the woman who was about to bear a child, that he might devour her child when she brought it forth" (Revelations 12:4). Hope, it is said, is giving birth in the face of the dragon. It is that impulse of hope that encourages us to go on despite the odds against our endeavor. It is that impulse of hope that sustained Anne Frank's belief that people are really good at heart even though she could "see the world gradually being turned into a wilderness . . . [and could] . . . feel the sufferings of millions." It is that impulse of hope that called on me to bear and bring forth a child despite the difficulties. Even in the harshest of poverty, the devastations of war, the threat of environmental annihilation, we continue to give birth, and each birth is an act of hope. We go on, not knowing whether or not we will succeed. We hope that we will, but hope is what refuses to fail us even if we fail.

Hope is an amazing thing. It does indeed seems to "spring eternal." I say I could not long exist without hope, in part because something in me refused to. In saying that, I mean not that something in me refused to exist if I were without hope, but rather that something in me refused to be without hope. There were days when I plunged into a well of despair so deep I thought I would drown in it. Then something would come along and lift me out. My hopeless times lasted only a few days at most. My spirit simply refused to give up its hope. Always something lifted it up. "Water within us, water surrounds us, a great mystery we grow dry at all." The waters of hope are always in us, always around us. A wellspring. "We go on . . . "

Where does it come from, this amazing wellspring of hope? After his statements about suffering producing hope, Paul goes on, "and hope does not disappoint us, because God's love has been poured into our hearts through the Holy Spirit which has been given to us" (Romans 5:4–5). Here Paul got it right. Love has been poured into our hearts. It is that love that produces hope, and hope that produces endurance.

In the days of waiting for the transplant, David often suggested that I prepare our son for the upcoming separation by doing practice separations. A few days and nights here and there of my being gone would ready him, toughen him up, produce endurance. No, no, I couldn't bear the thought. Who knows how many days I had ever to be with him, and then to leave him just to give him practice at my being gone? No. Rather, my impulse was just the opposite, to be with him as much as possible, to so fill him with my presence that in my absence he would not run dry but instead know the hope in his soul. I wanted to pour so much love into his soul that he could endure the vast spaces ahead. Love, presence, assurance—these, not suffering, produce hope. And when these are poured into one's heart and soul, suffering is endurable. We can go on when we are filled with the spirit's presence and love, when we are filled with each other's presence and love. I was so blessed with this.

Two things philosopher Hannah Arendt says are essential to our human existence: hope and faith—"a wing and a prayer." I suppose all of us who are waiting for transplants come to that day of deliverance— the day of the transplant itself—"on a wing and a prayer." Certainly I was sustained by the prayers of many, but for me, the final passage of this journey came on a kind of wing.

The LifeFlight helicopter flies over my house often; in those months of waiting I'd look up for it and wonder about its passengers. Who had they gone to rescue? Who were they delivering hope to today? When would it be my turn? Finally it was. Lifting off from the ground in the dark of that February night, taking a turn around the lake, soon to be delivered into freedom, I felt lifted in my hopes. These were angels, and this their chariot. "Swing low, sweet chariot, comin' for to carry me home." They were the deliverers of my hope. Guardian angels.

I still look to the sky when I hear chopper blades. Whose hope are they holding today?

There is a point in the play *The Diary of Anne Frank* where Anne has to go and see the sky. She cannot go another day without seeing it. It replenishes her spirit. "I hear the ever approaching thunder, which will destroy us too," she writes in her diary. "I can feel the sufferings of millions and yet, if I look up into the heavens, I think that it will all come right, that this cruelty too will end, and that peace and tranquility will return again."

I, too, tend to look skyward when in need of hope. The view from my window fills my heart with hope each day. I was drawn here by the view of the lake, but what I find myself watching now is the sky—sunrises, moonrises, rainbows, great cloud formations, the mists rising out of the valley, rays of light shining through the clouds, Orion, the Pleiades. All of these fill me with hope. Every morning and evening, just after the sunrise and just before sunset, gulls fly across the sky. They seem to lift me up with them. Hope is uplifting. As my eyes lift skyward so does my heart.

Hope is a testimony of the human spirit, always lifting us up, refusing to refuse us. I had said that suffering without hope kills the spirit, and perhaps I was wrong in that. Is anything so strong as to destroy that gift? More likely it is frozen or buried—like a bulb planted too deep or too shallow, yet always carrying a kernel of life inside. We are resilient.

Our spirits, and our hearts, are resilient. As Woody Allen said in one of his movies, "The heart is a resilient little muscle." Indeed. Never had I known such resiliency as this heart of mine, both my physical heart and my heart of hearts. Again and again, the forces of the universe commanded this heart to stop, and again and again it refused. Even as my own was stopped and cut out, in me was placed a new heart, with such hope—that this heart that had been cut from its home, that had stopped beating and had not beaten for several hours, that this heart would beat again. Think of it. They take this cold, still, lifeless lump of tissue, attach it to a warm body, let the warm blood flow, and then hope . . . hope that it will beat again. I can imagine no greater act of hope.

We go on . . . As this new heart brought hope to me, I imagine that in my going on, in our together going on, we carry the hopes of all my donor's loved ones as well. We go on . . . together.

We are a resilient people. We carry within us replenishing springs. We do go dry, but hope always replenishes.

Replenish, all must be replenished, . . . Replenish each shriveled heart . . . The heron's wing and the hope in our souls . . . we go on.

CLAUDIA SCHMIDT, "Replenish"

Patience

"Be patient toward all that is unsolved in your heart
and try to love the questions themselves . . .
the point is, to live everything. Live the questions now.
Perhaps you will then gradually, without noticing it,
live along some distant day into the answer."

RAINER MARIA RILKE

Be patient," counseled my mother as I sat squiggling and squirming in the "waiting" room of a doctor's office. There was little unsolved in my heart at the time, and the only question I really had was how much longer I would have to wait. "You need to learn to be patient," she said, and I remember being struck even then, at the age of eight or nine, by the joke of her telling me to be patient when there I was, being a patient. It is a joke often heard in the waiting areas of doctors' offices and clinics.

> Two people had been waiting to see the doctor for a very long time, and one began to complain to the other about how long they had been waiting. The other replied, "So, why do you think they call us 'patients'?"

Waiting. "Clients" wait in "reception areas"; "customers" in "customer service areas"—only "patients" wait in "waiting rooms." As patients we are expected to wait. The more critical patients are taken first. Emergencies happen. Doctors schedule more in a day than they can possibly do. Waiting is fundamental to our definition of "patients." Social workers, attorneys, and accountants see "clients"; clergy see "parishioners"; teachers see "students"; business people see "customers." Only health professionals—doctors, dentists, psychiatrists—see "patients." Several years ago there was a consumer movement to change our "title" from "patient" to "client" or "customer"—to recognize that patients are indeed paying customers and that our time is valuable. As such, patients should expect to be compensated for our wait, for time lost, time wasted; time is money after all. But it would be a mistake to make this change—first, in reducing the doctor/patient relationship to a cash nexus, but also in disguising the specific nature of the patient's waiting.

The waiting of a patient is different from the waiting of a customer or a client. A patient is not simply passing the time. A patient waiting to see a doctor is more often than not someone who is suffering. The patient is in distress, sick, in pain. It is one thing to wait for your car to be fixed when you're supposed to be at an appointment across town; quite another to wait for your broken leg to be set or your abscessed tooth to be drained. In our culture, adults have been socialized to hide our distress, to wait with decorum and silence. The true nature of the wait is found on the "peds" floor—the wailing, the crying, the coughing, the puking. These children are in pain; they are suffering—and they must wait.

The waiting of the sick person—for relief, for a cure, even for death, requires more than simply allowing time to pass. It is the endurance of suffering.

Waiting. As a patient I have done a lot of that. Waiting to see doctors. How often would we rush through Twin Cities traffic to be at the clinic at the designated hour, only to be told we'd have to wait to see the doctor. I have even been rushed by ambulance to get studies done "as soon as possible"—only to have the studies postponed for several days. There was waiting for test results and for insurance company approval and of course, the longest and hardest wait—for the heart itself. Every transplant patient I have met has said it is the waiting that is the hardest.

It's interesting to watch my moods change from day to day. A few days ago I was in absolute despair. Yesterday I woke up cynical and apathetic. Today I am anxious. I'm not sure why. I am both fearful that the transplant won't come in time, and hopeful that it will. . . .

They're right. This waiting is the hardest.

AUGUST 23, 1993

Some people are told they need a transplant immediately, and they receive it in a week or a month. They are spared the wait, though I imagine this has its own hardships. But most wait long—months, years. Many transplant patients spend their days of waiting in the hospital, often in intensive care. Some who relocate to be nearer to the transplant center spend months and years away from home, family, and friends. I was lucky. I was able to be in my own home. I was able to continue to work. I rarely saw the inside of a hospital. There were days, even weeks, when the waiting was easy, hardly a test of my patience.

For me, the testing of my patience was directly related to the suffering I was called upon to endure. When my rhythm was stable, I would be content for the call to be delayed as long as possible, but when my rhythm was bad . . .

I have been so lucky to have lived such a normal life to this point. Otherwise, I don't know how I could have survived the waiting so far. Right now every day seems an eternity. Will I make it through another day?

The phone rings—I hope it is my heart. I used to be scared at the thought of that phone call. Now I am eager for it. I imagine the call coming and just saying, "Thank you. Thank you."

AUGUST 8, 1993

Patience for me was not about days of stability. Patience was about getting through evenings of uncertainty, when the rhythm was so bad that I thought surely I would explode or die. Patience was about sitting in church or in movie theaters or in department meetings, feeling my heart beat, listening to it pound, all the time wondering if I would be shocked. Patience was about sitting by the window watching my little boy play in the snow—longing to be out there with him, unable to be with him, aching to be with him. Patience was about all those days in the hospital away from Paul.

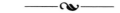

It is a beautiful day. The sun is shining; the air is clear. The lake and sky are deep shades of blue. But I am looking at them from a hospital bed again.

Oh my dear Paul, I am so sad to leave you again. How I miss being home with you.

TO PAUL, JULY 4, 1990

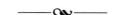

Here I am in a hospital bed again. The ache I feel in missing you is matched only by thinking of the kind of pain of separation you must be feeling. How I hate to think of you hurting. I miss you so.

TO PAUL, FEBRUARY 24, 1991

Here I am again, writing to you from a hospital bed . . .

It is a beautiful day and I just want to be home and playing with you. . . .

I can hardly stand this separation. . . . How I long to rock you to sleep, to hold you in my arms, to hear you say "Mommy come." I want to come home and be your mommy.

TO PAUL, JUNE 4, 5, and 6, 1991

Patience was about one summer after the next of not camping, not canoeing, not swimming, not journeying to Michigan to visit my family.

———— ❧ ————

I have said "next summer" so many times. This is the third summer of waiting. And next summer, will I still be saying "next summer?"

It is difficult to believe in anymore.

AUGUST 24, 1993

Patience was about one beautiful fall after another of not being out hiking. "Oh, may I go a-wandering, until the day I die. . . ." Paul would play the song over and over, and every time I thought, "Yes, may I go a-wandering. I want to go a-wandering until I die. That's how I want to die, out there, hiking in the hills, not in here waiting by the phone or lying in some hospital bed." Patience was about telling Paul over and over again, "I can't . . . I can't . . . When I get my new heart."

There were agonies of pain, fear, fatigue, incapacity, all of which tested my patience, but perhaps the greatest test of my patience, as well as that of everyone around me, was enduring the agonizing of my mind and heart. Had I made the right decision? Should I go ahead with the transplant? Should I stop this whole process now?

"Be patient toward all that is unsolved in your heart," counseled the quote from Rainer Maria Rilke that hangs over my desk. There was so much that was unsolved in my heart. The disease was unsolved. What to do about the disease was unsolved.

"Live the questions," Rilke continues. I lived the questions daily, and they tested my patience, and I imagine the patience of all the caregivers—nurses, doctors, my family, friends—who patiently listened and responded to my many questions and doubts. In Hermann Hesse's *Siddartha*, Siddartha remarks on how the river "was always the same and yet every moment it was new." So were my questions. Like the repeated "When will we get there?" of my child, and the twentieth repetition of the same question of my 88-year-old grandmother, for whom the same questions appeared always new, so now did my questions appear to me. The same questions appeared to my mind over and over, usually in the middle of the night, and yet each time they presented themselves to me as if they were new. To be patient is to endure the questions over and over, again and again. To read through my journals from that time is to go round and round the question—always with different answers.

———— ❧ ————

I have been going round and round all night about whether to go ahead with the transplant.

APRIL 29, 1992

———— ❧ ————

I don't want a transplant.

SEPTEMBER 19, 1992

———— ❧ ————

Am I trading one form of infirmity for another? That is the unanswerable question that has been rumbling around my brain for days.

Right now, I can't go hiking in the hills or running on the beach. I can't dance my heart out or dive into a cool lake. I can't drive myself any farther than the confines of this town. I can't hop a plane to see my sister. I can make love only passively, not passionately. I can make life only passively, not passionately.

But I can walk. I can see. I can hold my baby in my arms. I can care for him when he is sick. Though my heart is critically ill, I feel in relatively good health. And who knows, I may survive a long time.

My question is, might I be putting these simple yet extraordinary pleasures of life at risk in pursuit of those others? In wanting to hike, might I lose the ability to walk? In wanting to see my sister might I lose my sight? Am I asking for too much? Should I just rest content, learning to live with these limitations, preferable to others that might arise after the transplant?

SEPTEMBER 26, 1992

————— ❦ —————

I feel so well, the thought of cutting out my heart seems senseless. I know there have been so many times I thought I wouldn't make it through the day, let alone the year. Right now, I feel I could live out a normal life span. . . .
It is so hard to know what to do.

OCTOBER 10, 1992

————— ❦ —————

The decision is made. It feels clear.
And I am relieved. The seesaw of wondering is over.

OCTOBER 19, 1992

————— ❦ —————

Here I am in a quandary again . . .

FEBRUARY 23, 1994

I needed to learn patience. How to endure suffering. How to endure the waiting and the wondering, the terror and the torture, the incapacity and the indecision . . . and not crack, and not break, and not burst in anger and violence. These are the lessons of patience, for the patience of the endurance of suffering is not simply about the endurance itself, but about the manner in which the suffering is endured. To endure suffering patiently means to endure it silently, steadfastly, without complaint, anger, and irritability. But something bothers me about this. It causes me to conjure up images of the battered wife silently enduring abuse without complaint; of oppressed peoples quiescently accepting the injustices of their lives. It makes patience out to be passivity and defeatism in the face of oppression.

I don't think of patience as being a passive quality, but rather an active presence of steadfast calm and assurance; an affirmative quality, one that uplifts and affirms the soul, not one that is defeated. When I think of patience, what comes to mind is Reinhold Niebuhr's "serenity prayer":

> God grant me the ability to accept the things I cannot change,
> the courage to change the things I can,
> and the wisdom to know the difference.

All of these—changing the things we can, accepting the things we can't change, and wisely knowing the difference between the two—are part of an active patience. Patience requires that we change the things we can. As much as patience is the endurance of suffering, it is also the seeking of change. A patient is not someone who is passively accepting their suffering as their lot in life, but someone who seeks relief from that suffering, who in a way that is affirming of their being seeks to change their situation to the extent that they can. A patient is someone who is seeking the counsel and aid of a physician, who can help to bring about the desired change in their lives. For me, patience did not demand that I simply endure the condition of my life. Rather, patience demanded that I seek to change everything I could. I meditated and went through holistic therapy; I underwent surgery to implant a defibrillator; I tried medication after medication; and ultimately I sought to change my very heart itself. It was only when I had exhausted my options, when finally I had nothing left but to wait for the heart, that I could begin the process of patiently waiting my turn (though there were still the meanderings of my mind to contend with).

At that point, patience was a matter of letting go. Having done all that could be done, I simply had to trust in the rest. I couldn't change the damage done to my heart. I couldn't speed up my place in line. I needed to be patient with the process. Nor could I stop my questioning. My questions had a process of their own, and I needed to be as patient with my own process as with the process of the transplant. What did it mean to be patient with my process, with the process? To accept these necessities of being a transplant patient, to accept this need, I had to question and not try to hurry it along. Patience is to be without haste—to let the answer find its own time, to let the fruit ripen on the vine. "You can't push a river," sings Margie Adam. The heart would come in its own time, as would the answers to my questions.

For some questions there are no answers until we arrive.

"When will we get there?" cries the child every ten minutes of the ride. When we are there. "When will this be over?" asked a friend of mine in childbirth. When the baby comes. "When will this waiting be over?" I query. When the heart comes. In my days of waiting, my friend Jean counseled me to trust—trust that the universe was finding just the right heart for me, and I knew she was talking about more than the physical qualities of blood and tissue type. Trust in the universe. Patience requires letting go.

As it requires mindfulness—an appreciation of the present moment. The words of Dan Millman, author of *Way of the Peaceful Warrior*, kept repeating in my mind, reminding me to stay in the present:

> *"Where are you?"*
> *"Here."*
> *"What time is it?"*
> *"Now."*

DAN MILLMAN, *Way of the Peaceful Warrior*

To be mindful is to be ever aware that the time and place are here and now. There is no need to ask when we will get there, for we are in the here and now. The impatient cry of "When will we get there?" is the cry of a child focused on the destination, rather than the journey. I was most impatient with the time of waiting when I was sure of the transplant decision. At those times I would focus on the destination, and how soon I would get there, rather than the journey itself.

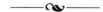

My heart rhythm is bad again, and there seems no end in sight. I worry that this heart transplant will not happen in my lifetime. My patience is running thin.

JULY 28, 1992

In many ways, my questioning of the transplant decision helped make me more patient with the waiting. All my questioning of *whether* I wanted this particular destination or not helped my impatience about *when* I was getting there. My questioning focused my attention on my present quandary. I was not hurrying to a particular destination. The questions helped me to live one day at a time, indeed, one moment at a time. The counsel to live "one day at a time" speaks of mindfulness, a focusing on the present rather than the future. Fully focused on the present, impatience for the future disappears.

Mindfulness is appreciation of the present moment. But how does one appreciate the present moment when it is filled with suffering? There may come a time when suffering is so intense and so constant that one's spirit is broken. Certainly, had the bouts of shocking gone on incessantly, my patience and spirit would have rapidly died. Most suffering, the suffering I have known, has its intermittencies, like labor pains, which are bearable in part because of the spaces between contractions.

I am reminded again of Sisyphus, who day after day rolls his rock up the mountain, only to have it roll back down. Sisyphus turns, goes back down and rolls it up again. He doesn't collapse in defeat at the top and refuse to descend, saying, "I can't. I can't." He pauses for a moment, and then patiently turns and picks up his rock again. He simply does what needs to be done. Patience requires this ability to pick up and go on, to overcome disappointment, not to give up in defeat. Philosopher Albert Camus says that one must imagine Sisyphus happy. That has always struck me as strange. Then I think of the Buddhist practice of the half-smile, which encourages consciously smiling to nourish the inner calm of mindfulness. Perhaps

Sisyphus is smiling because he has made peace with his rock—neither defeating it nor being defeated by it. We can't change everything, but we can change what we can and make peace with the rest. Our rocks may roll down the mountain again and again, but they need not crush us.

With every setback, every shock, every six-month repetition of the prediction, "It'll be in the next six months," every winter every summer every spring every fall come and gone, every bout of ectopy, my rock rolled down the mountain. There were times I endured it patiently. There were times I just wanted to lie down and quit, to say I can't do this anymore. I had been pushed beyond patience to defeat. Then something would pick me up, and I could turn again and carry yet another rock up the mountain. That something was hope.

Thus did I find that patience does not spring forth on its own, but rather requires all these others—faith, trust, letting go, mindfulness, hope—to give it birth and sustenance. Given these, patience will come. When will patience come? In its own time.

"If you wait, God will manifest Himself. Of course, you may have a long wait," writes Cistercian monk Thomas Keating. I had waited long for an answer to my questions and for a new heart. And then the day and the answer came. "We have a heart for you," said Sofia. My mind was swirling. Is this the right thing to do? Shouldn't we discuss this one more time? And then it was clear. I had, as Rilke suggested, lived along some distant day into the answer.

Generosity and receiving

———— ❧ ————

One thing that has impressed me throughout has been the generosity and good will of so many—even of relative strangers. So many people sincerely and willingly offering their help. Mary at the vet's offering to take care of Sam. Toni, the nurse practitioner, offering her children's baby-sitting services. Dave's Aunt Betty offering her home. The many who have offered to drive David or take care of Paul or do whatever needs to be done. And literally the hundreds who offer up prayers for me every day. How could I not be humbled and filled with gratitude. Of all the good things to come of this, I am so struck by the generous spirit of humanity.

OCTOBER 20, 1992

The outpouring—of love, of prayer, of sustenance of body and spirit—came immediately. I was unaware of most of it—the doctors and nurses who poured their wisdom, skill, hope, and literally their breath into my body; the many women from the coffeehouse who kept vigil outside my hospital room; the neighbors who brought food; a friend barely known to David who walked him through this initial crisis with a calm and steady hand; my sister who came at a moment's notice. On a conscious level, I knew nothing of these, but on a deeper level, I know that these gifts wrapped me in warm blankets of love and carried me through on prayerful hope. When I first awoke from the arrest, my sensations were of being held by hundreds of gentle, loving arms and of being bathed in a light of soothing soft whiteness—the palpable presence of the prayers of all those who had sustained me through the first horrific hours and days.

The generosity extended far beyond that moment of crisis. In the long sieges that lay ahead, the generosity was unending. It is said that difficult times bring out the best and the worst in people. I was continually shown the best of humanity. I was so blessed by kindnesses large and small—the genuine heartfelt concern, a marked gentleness and patience and support. But I was most struck by the generosity of actions and efforts and spirit.

So many people wanted to help, to give of themselves. Immediately following the first cardiac arrest, dozens sent cards and flowers and good wishes. Food arrived at the house; friends arrived at the hospital. The women of the coffeehouse not only held vigil outside my hospital room, they also organized a "social services" network among the membership for me, which included not only a "meals on wheels" program, but also cleaning, childcare, gardening, massage. I was well and generously taken care of. They were family to me.

In the following weeks and months, friends brought books and videos and music and other precious gifts—roses from their garden, a spring bouquet of wildflowers picked along the roadside, a healing crystal found on Lake Superior's North Shore. Yet more precious to me than any of these was simply the fact that people came. Their presence, their willingness literally to "be there" for me, touched me so deeply.

Some came when they could; some came even when they couldn't. And when those who wanted to really couldn't, they called. While she could rarely be here, my friend Judy would call from wherever in the world she was—Beijing, China; Novy Sacz, Poland; Zagreb, Croatia. They came to be near even in my hours of unconsciousness. They came to support David in his hours of need. They came—gathering round, like the lovers in Pete Seeger's song "Old Devil Time"—and helped me rise to fight this one more time.

Some came to cheer me and be of good company. When I could not travel, family, friends, and former students and teachers made the extra effort to come to me. At times, there was a sense that they were coming to pay their last respects. I had done that with my mother and my father and knew that there is a tone, an intentionality to that last visit. I am sure many came thinking it might be the last time. But this did not seem morbid to me. It was reality. I was grateful for this chance to be with them one last time.

Some of these visits were especially touching. Among them was that of my high school choir director and his wife. He had been like a father to me in my high school days. Now, in his seventy-somethings, when by all rights I should be making the effort to come visit him, he and his wife traveled two thousand miles across country to spend some time with me. We caught up on each others' lives and reminisced and played duets on the piano. In my memory those duets play like Pooh's "sustaining songs."

Then there were Barb and Sam, a former student and her friend. In the early days following my arrest, when it was not prudent for Paul to be alone with me, they had come for a couple weeks simply to be a presence in our home. When they were married the next summer, I was too sick to travel to their wedding, so they gave up some of their honeymoon time to come be with us.

Some came to give comfort and care—for me, for David, and for Paul. My sister-in-law Wanda came at a time when my rhythm got so bad I could no longer care for Paul by myself. She cared for us and cooked for us and took us to the beach and the park and read *Go, Dog, Go* to Paul over and over until he could recite the entire book back to us. Her reassuring presence helped calm my heart and helped us feel safe and secure until we could feel that way on our own again.

In the months following my last shocking episode, when I had been shocked lying in bed, I didn't feel safe anywhere. My heart rhythm had so deteriorated, I no longer felt secure being alone with Paul, and I certainly didn't feel that I should be driving. During that time, Dave's dad came and stayed with us off and on. He was our chauffeur and sometimes tended our garden. As with Wanda, his simply being here was the greatest gift, helping us to feel more at ease, and Paul was so happy to have his grandpa here for awhile.

My friend and former student Genni came to see me each time I was in the University Hospital, but the time I remember most was a few days after the transplant. I was feeling particularly blue, and I worried about Paul and David so far away in Duluth. In the midst of a Minnesota winter, she walked into my room with armloads of fresh watermelon and peaches and grapes. I hardly remember the words that passed between us. I only remember that she was just the person I needed to be with, that she said just what I needed to hear, that her presence was so very healing to me, and that I felt held in such comfort.

My friend Jody, who had been a regular presence at my bedside with every hospitalization, came to care for me in Minneapolis for a few days after my transplant. She cooked wonderful meals (though my system couldn't quite handle the tofu yet!), gave me backrubs, and quite literally brought me the moon and stars to glow in the dark above my bed at night. She got me out of the house and into the fresh air of those first warm days of early March. I basked in the sunshine of her good cheer.

And of course there was my sister, Jeannie. I have lost track of the number of times she came. Suffice it to say, our spare bedroom has become known as "Aunt Jeannie's room." She made us meals and did our laundry and spent hours upon hours with Paul—reading stories, blowing bubbles, lining up plastic animals in parades, building card-table caves. She brought her family to cheer our Christmas holidays. She kept David good company in his crisis times and in his early morning coffee times. She rubbed my feet for hours to distract me from the pain following surgery. And for six weeks after the transplant, she cared for me. One of the criteria that must be met to qualify for a heart transplant is some one person who is committed to your care. I couldn't have done it without her. She went to the grocery store, cooked my meals, washed the dishes in the laundry tub at Aunt Betty's, made me cups of hot tea, drove me to the clinic nearly every day for tests or rehabilitation, comforted me in my middle-of-the-night pains, scraped the ice off the car windows and drove me to the emergency room on the one night we had bad weather, put up with all my complaints and fears and prednisone irritability, and generally kept me good company. Who else could I have felt so comfortable with in my moans and groans and fears and dependency? In the months before the transplant, when it seemed I might never get a heart, she often said she wished she could give me her heart. The fact is, she did.

Some came in moments of crisis. In 1990, as I awaited heart surgery for the first time in my life, my surgeon brother flew out to be with me. I felt safer knowing he was there. Four years later, both my brothers flew to Minneapolis on the day of the transplant. I had asked them both to come, and they did. Thinking of that time now, my request seems a little silly, since I was unconscious most of the time they were there and have little memory of their presence. But simply knowing they would be there helped get me through my fears and apprehensions surrounding the operation. I suppose it is like learning how to ride a bicycle or how to swim. You can do it on your own if you have to, but knowing that a hand is there to steady your ride or hold you up on the surface makes the deed seem more doable. Before the transplant, knowing they would come helped me enter the water, and afterward, knowing they had come helped me to swim. I felt so held.

More support came from my nephew Mark. He had always said he was planning on coming for the transplant, and indeed he did. He stayed for several days and was a great source of companionship for David. But mostly he was there for me, eager to care for me—he even suctioned out my ventilator tubes—and to protect me, sleeping each night in my hospital room. I often wonder what I have done to elicit the generous love of this young man, that he would fly out for my operation and spend every day and night by my side.

In the intervening years, between my first arrest and the transplant, I faced several smaller moments of crisis. For these our friends gathered round. One day, shortly after returning home after my first arrest, I suddenly was in tachycardia again. David was not home, so one friend drove me to the emergency room while others cared for Paul.

Another night, not long after my second arrest, I went into tachycardia quite suddenly while watching a movie. We called Jerry, Paul's pediatrician who lives next door, to be with us, just in case I arrested again. Rather than supplying CPR, he guided me through a meditation of warm sunshine filling my body. Soon my heart slowed and was calm.

And then there is Nancy. What good fortune that our dear neighbor across the street is not only the most giving person I have met, but a coronary care nurse. For nearly four years, she laid out her clothes beside her bed each night in the event that I would need her, as I often did. She was always there. Always there. In countless ways. She held me through the shocking. She took me to the late-night visits to the emergency room. My first day back teaching, she sat in my office across the hall, just in case something should go wrong. She stayed with me the entire day of my heart catherization for my transplant work-up. She stayed with Paul when David drove me to the helicopter for my transplant. In my nights of fear, she slept on our couch. On the worst nights, she slept in my bed. I just wanted her near. I felt so safe and comforted by her presence. It seems that even now, if anything goes wrong in our lives, even if it's a bad dream, my first thought is "Call Nancy!"

Some cared for me by caring for Paul. Annie, Paul's first real baby-sitter, was a blessing in our lives. When I was stuck in a hospital and needing help, she offered hers. She has been such a tender presence to both Paul and me.

When Paul was three and a half, he went to day care, which we simply called "Lynn's." How could I have made it through without Lynn? Her father had just undergone a kidney transplant, so she had a better understanding of what I was facing than just about anyone. She became Paul's "other mother." She was ready, willing, and able to care for him anytime. She was especially good at helping Paul deal with his fears and questions and feelings. When I had to be gone all those weeks after the transplant, I could rest assured that he was in good and loving hands. How could I have left him so long in anyone else's care?

Except of course his Aunt Cyd's, Dave's sister. She took care of Paul for us so many times, especially during the times surrounding my arrests. During those two weeks immediately following the transplant, when David couldn't be home with him, she lovingly took Paul in. And I could be sure that he was getting all the love and understanding he needed to get him through that rough time. It was just such a gift to me that I could go into the transplant knowing that he had such loving hands to hold him in our absence.

We not only had a home for Paul, we had a home for our dog, Sam. Any time we left town on an emergency, and when we left for the transplant, our neighbors Jean and Jerry took Sam in, and I could rest assured that he too had a loving home. Sometimes I think my absence was harder on him than on anyone else. He didn't know why I left . . . why our walks stopped. Of everyone, he always seemed the most glad to see me when I returned home. He is a gift to me too. What a pure presence of love.

And I had a home. For months I had been distraught over what I was going to do for housing in Minneapolis during the three months I needed to be there following the transplant. There was the Kidney House, a boarding house for transplant patients, and that would have been fine for me, but not for Paul. We needed a place where we could be a family. We thought of renting an apartment, but what could we find in one week right after the transplant? And how could we afford that? Where could we go? Where could we go? I stayed up nights pondering that question, churning it over in my stomach. We began to think of people we knew in Minneapolis. I had good friends there, but none with much room. And it seemed like such a huge request—to take in someone recovering from a heart transplant and her family. How could I ask anyone to do that? I did ask a couple of people, and they expressed their willingness, but then Dave's Aunt Betty generously offered us the perfect solution. She had a downstairs bedroom/living area we could have for the duration. It was just twenty minutes from the hospital, in a quiet area, with a playground for Paul. This was ideal. I cannot begin to convey the relief of that burden being lifted from my shoulders the day she offered her home to us. Her generosity made the transplant so much easier. One of the most difficult aspects of facing the transplant was looking at all those months away from home. Now we had a home to go to. For six weeks she opened her home to us, and her home became ours. Such a gift.

My colleagues were equally generous and allayed another of my greatest concerns, losing my job. So many people lose their jobs while awaiting transplant, and one of the hardest things for them to deal with after the transplant is that loss of employment. I am so fortunate to have been able to work up to the last hours before my transplant, and then come back to it afterwards. My colleagues took care of me as if they were family. There were two weeks left in the quarter when I first arrested in 1990, and various members of the faculty picked up my courses and carried them on for me, including the hardest part, the final grading. Fortunately, I had arranged for a sabbatical for the following year, so that was not a problem. I had that year off to heal, or so I thought. My condition was stable, and my meds somewhat straightened out, but I did not heal. By the following year, I didn't know if I could survive the classroom or not. I was frightened that the strain— or the passion—of teaching would get my heart pumping so fast that it would slip into tachycardia; I would be shocked, or arrest; and I knew that there would not be nurses and doctors on hand in that audience of students (though later one of the students told me she had been trained as an emergency medical technician and reassured me that I could count on her). My department and college generously gave me reduced loads, smaller classes, and fewer committee assignments, all of which enabled me to work through all of this. My department even arranged to have all my classes next to the department office so that someone could be there in case of an emergency. I am quite certain that one of my colleagues came to work early on those days that I had 7:45 classes, just to be sure someone was around if I needed help. They were all so good to me. The students were generous and understanding as well, and genuinely concerned.

Then there were those who listened patiently to my wonderings and woes. My friends and family certainly did that, but I think particularly of my doctor here in Duluth and all of the people associated with the transplant program. They listened to my questions over and over. Should I have the transplant or not? What does this symptom mean? What if this happens? Where am I on the list now? I always felt listened to. I always felt they would take as much time with me as I needed. They were so generous with their time and patience.

And my minister listened. She walked through this with me. She listened to my fears, and I could talk with her about the very real prospect of my death, something I couldn't talk about with many people. We talked about my memorial service and how the church would help support David and Paul through their grief. And she was just regularly there for me. I imagine she knew it would be important to my healing to share my experience, and it was she who first suggested I explore the spiritual aspects of my transplant as a vehicle for that process. This book is in many ways her continuing gift of listening to me.

Finally, David. He gave fully to me, without resentment. The generosity of his love came pouring out. Anything, anything he could do . . . all the trips to Minneapolis, the visits to the hospital, the middle-of-the-night comforts, the back rubs, the games of cribbage and Trouble that distracted me from my anxieties . . . all the fishing trips he gave up . . . all the time with his family . . . all the time for his work. I look back on it now with such fondness, especially that first week at Aunt Betty's after the transplant. We moved easily together. He cooked for me, bathed me, cared for me, and genuinely seemed to enjoy it all. We watched old Mary Tyler Moore reruns, and he played solitaire while I slept. We were precious to each other. Such generosity he gave me. He gave up his time; he gave up his dreams for a time; he gave up his life—and gave it up gladly.

I can't name all the names. So many gave me rides, food, flowers; planted my garden; walked my dog; cleaned my house. And I can't name all the names because there are so many I don't even know. At times it is the generosity of these strangers that touches me the most. I think of the generosity of the people who kept me alive—doctors and nurses who came out of the audiences, who kept me alive with their bodies and their breath; the paramedics—some of whom I have been able to thank, but most of whom remain nameless; the emergency room nurses and doctors, the coronary care nurses. I owe my very life to these people, and I don't even know their names. Hundreds of people who witnessed my arrests came to the hospital, sent cards and flowers and well wishes. Literally hundreds of people, mostly unknown to me, prayed for me—the prayer chain at our church, the prayer chain at my sister's church, the prayer chain at my nephew's college, indeed his whole campus community.

That people offered their prayers so generously, in all varieties of forms, was overwhelming to me. The women of the coffeehouse sent healing energy that embraced me as I awoke the first time in University Hospital. David's grandmother lit a candle for me every day. A spiritualist friend of my sister spent an hour every day sending me light. And every morning David would walk to our wedding spot in the woods and say a prayer for me. So much energy, so generously given, and so often by people whom I did not even know.

So much, so very much. As I go through this litany of generosity—this incredible overflowing of spirit—I am still overwhelmed to the point of tears.

In the first phases of my journey through all of this, when I was both in and out of this world, I was open to it all. How it sustained me. It was only later that I began to have difficulty with it. As I grew more cognizant and aware, as I returned to my home and the guardedness of my private life and personal autonomy, I found it difficult to receive all that was poured out to me. I had been reared to be self-sufficient and fairly private. I could ask for help from my family, but no one else. Now I needed lots of help from all quarters. It was hard to ask. It was harder still to receive. It may be more blessed to give than to receive; for some of us, it's also easier.

I'm not sure why I was so resistant to receiving the gifts people offered so generously. Perhaps it was that I didn't want to be someone who simply took from people. There are, it seems to me, some people who give and give and give and some who just take, who suck you dry of anything you have to give. I didn't want to be a taker. Perhaps it was pride, not wanting to show my weakness, my vulnerability, my very real need—"the visibility without which we cannot truly live." Perhaps it was that three-year-old "me do" spark of autonomy that insists on total self-reliance. Perhaps it was part of that armoring, that left-over unopened heart, that didn't want to let others in—their gifts, their songs, their love, their lives. A guarding, an armor.

What ultimately made it easier to receive all these generous spirits into my life was something I had read in my perusal of the literature on healing—that generosity, the giving of gifts, is very healing to the one who gives. To allow someone to give to me then was really giving something to them. I suppose receiving with an attitude of generosity is different from taking simply to get all you can get. At least it enabled me to receive. To receive graciously, thankfully, is a real gift to the many people who are so hungry to give. So often our society seems so Hobbesian—we are so afraid of being taken that we take first. Yet it is this taking and fear of being taken, wasting away our energies on one-upmanship, keeping up, fighting for our place in line, that leaves us with nothing left to give. And that is what really dries us up—having no time or energy left to give. I have seen how deep in the spirit of humanity is this spirit of generosity and how it does indeed fill our wells.

A Buddhist proverb about heaven and hell says that, in both, people are seated at a great feast, with twelve-foot-long chopsticks. In hell, they try to feed themselves. In heaven, they feed each other. It seems that this circle of generous giving and receiving is heaven indeed.

I had been given to over and over again, but there was one last gift I had yet to receive, the greatest gift, again the gift of a stranger, the gift of the heart itself. Waiting for the heart, that is, waiting for someone to die so that I could live, was so odd, so very difficult. I knew all the realities of how my waiting for the heart had nothing to do with their death, that no one was being sacrificed for me, that nothing was being bought or sold. This person would have died anyway. Nevertheless, I did feel something of a vulture, waiting for the death that would sustain me. That my life depended on the death of another was one of the hardest aspects of all of this. How does one prepare to receive the heart of another—the life of another—especially when that other is a child, and I knew that given my size, it most likely would be the heart of a child. How can one receive such a gift?

I suppose the receiving of the generous gifts of so many before the transplant had helped prepare me, helped open my heart. Each gift helped open me to receive this greatest gift of life.

Preparing for that gift was also helped by my earlier discovery—

113

that being able to give to someone is so very healing. I could only hope that in my graciously receiving this heart I would be helping in the healing of someone's grief—that we could somehow feed each other at this banquet of life and death.

In *A Gift from the Sea*, Anne Morrow Lindbergh writes of how purposeless giving depletes us, whereas purposeful giving is restorative. I have heard this from many donor families, that the giving of their loved one's organs transforms a purposeless death into a purposeful gift, and in that transformation all are healed.

My donor and her family are strangers to me no longer. And their generosity to me continues. They have been so generous with their stories and with their own gratitude that their loved one lives on to a certain extent in me. Their gift of life to me in their loved one's heart continues to sustain my life every moment of every day. Their gifts of generous spirit make the receiving gentler.

Generosity. The Ojibwe consider it the most important quality in their leaders. The greatness of one's spirit—one's power—is revealed not in how much one can take charge, but rather in how generously one gives of one's life.

I have been so overwhelmed by the power of that generosity.

And I have been called upon to generously receive and have learned that it is indeed a gift to receive, and receive graciously, with an open heart. There is a generosity, a graciousness of receiving—a gracious gratitude, neither apologetic nor critical, simply accepting with an open heart. I think of the Christmas I made incredibly ugly, though I fancied them lovely, sequined cork earrings for my mother. I remember her genuine delight upon receiving them and then her generously wearing them to church that day. Such a gift that was to me. There can be a generosity in receiving.

Perhaps the greatest generosity of all is indeed in receiving—receiving others into one's life, whatever their gifts may be. The gifts may not be what you expect, nor even what you want, but the generosity lies in being open to them just them same. To accept with an open heart, to receive with gracious gratitude.

Gratitude

———— ◌ ————

*Today I ventured up into my sacred place. It is a spot high
up on the hills of Hawk Ridge, nestled among the pines, tucked
into the hillside, yet wide open to the sky and to the lake, which
stretches out beneath. I come here to find myself, to touch and
be touched by the universe. I have not been here for some time.
It has been too risky to wander in these woods, to climb these
heights. Today I came home. As I entered the sanctuary of pines,
I wept. Wept in gratitude—for this new heart, for the privilege
of being in this place once again. I wept throughout my climb.
Wept for this child whose heart I carry, whose heart carries
me. Wept for the family whose loss I bear, whose loss bears me.
I am so grateful to be alive.*

MAY 1994

Gratitude did not come easily nor immediately to me in all of
this. One might have thought that upon waking up from a
cardiac arrest that I narrowly survived, I would have been
filled with gratitude for being alive. But I wasn't. At that time, I really
was not cognizant of the edge I was on. I had no memory of the arrest
and the pursuant trauma and tenuousness. All I knew was that my life
had been rudely interrupted, my baby was far away, and I wanted to

115

go home and get on with my life. I was determined that life would go on as usual.

But life was not "usual" after that. My new life was a nightmare. Repeatedly shocked, snatched from my home into the clutches of coronary care, struggling with medication dosages that made my heart variously calm and tormented—this was not the life I had envisioned. This was not the life I wanted.

I was angry.

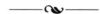

I am so angry today. Angry at having my life stripped away from me. Angry at living in such uncertainty, with such constraint on my actions and choices. Angry at doctors who don't have time to listen. Angry at having to fill my body/mind with pills—pills to counteract the effects of other pills. Angry at whatever forces have brought me to this place. . . .

Sweet Juniper [my dog who had died a year before]. *The other night I dreamt that you were going to pull me out of the water through the hole in the ice. But once I was under, the ice formed back over the hole before you could get to me. . . . Are you trying to get me through to your side of the universe? Or are you trying to pull me back to life? . . .*

Paul pulls me back to earth. But loving this life is hard when it seems so fragile and transient . . . and so I am angry.

SEPTEMBER 16, 1990

My journal entries of that time are filled with words like "robbed" and "cheated." I was robbed of my time with my son in those early months and years when he was changing so quickly and every moment is precious. I was cheated out of a life that was finally, after depths of grief and arduous struggle, what I wanted it to be.

Slowly, gradually, the space of my life narrowed down to a fraction of what it had been. I was stripped of my freedoms and my joys one by one, down to the bare bones of my existence. My baby was snatched from my breast before we had finished. My breasts swelled and ached, and I grew feverish for him, but it was over before either of us was ready. Nor could I hold him and calm his fears, for he no longer trusted me not to disappear and could find no comfort in these suspect arms. He was angry too, angry at me for leaving him—the one thing I had vowed I would never do, and yet it was done. I was angry about that.

My driver's license was revoked, and in this society to do that is to deprive a person of their freedom of movement. I remember the day my father took away his father's driver's license because he was no longer fit to drive and how they both cried at this final slash at his autonomy. I remembered as well how I was too afraid of demeaning my father to take away his driver's license and how I wished I had; now my mother was dead because I hadn't. Now I was being demeaned and diminished and my world denied, but I also knew that I was a danger on the highways.

And certain things were dangers to me. The list of endangering and endangered activities grew. Walking in the woods, working in the garden, speaking in public, carrying my child, engaging in a passionate discussion—all of these became dangerous to me. I had arrested while giving a piano performance; I had arrested engaging in political discourse; I had been shocked while I was digging in my garden; I had even gone into tachycardias watching a suspenseful movie and reading an emotionally powerful book. I was an endangered woman. Endangered because all that was me and mine was at risk of becoming extinct. In the process, I was losing my self. Yes, I was deprived of my freedoms—to have children, to teach, to travel, to walk and run and swim and ski and skate and hike and dance . . . But more than this, I was deprived of my life source, my touchpoint with my soul—the capacity to feel anything deeply.

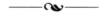

I have been forced to abandon the erotic. . . . The hours in the woods are gone. No longer can I immerse my body in the waters of Lake Superior. My body cannot move in joyous dance. Nor can I speak passionately my beliefs and concerns. Instead my life is carefully monitored by this least erotic of devices, a

computer. Caution and rationality have replaced passion and abandon in my being.

NOVEMBER 5, 1991

It seemed I was being deprived of life itself. I resented my deprivations, and the resentment was eating me alive. Albert Camus talks about resentment as autointoxication—self-poisoning. This is indeed what I was doing, poisoning myself by focusing my attention on all of the things I could not do. "I can't . . . I can't . . . I can't . . . " was my familiar refrain. "Refrain from this; refrain from that . . . ," until the refrain became the refrainment itself, boxing in my spirit as surely as this box in my chest did my body. I literally could not continue in the pursuit of every thought of what was wrong with my life. As trite and Pollyanaish as it might sound, I had to come to some insight about what was valuable in this. I had to come to see the blessedness of this event in my life. I *had* to. Not because of some syrupy "should," but because it was necessary for my survival, for my well-being.

So for the sake of my spiritual, emotional, and physical survival, I began to look for the blessing in the curse. From this grew a sense of gratitude. Gratitude got me through the resentment.

Among the blessings I discovered was a unique opportunity to gain perspective into the lives of others whose lives I would not otherwise have known. I felt I had a somewhat better, though limited, view of what it is to suffer the oppression of being poor or black in this country, simply by knowing what it was to be stripped of one's life choices. Granted, no *one* was pressing down on me. No *one* was trying to belittle, humiliate, or intentionally deprive me of my freedom and dignity. Nevertheless, I was able to witness something of what it is to have one's life's choices severely limited.

I knew a bit of the horror of living in a war zone. At least my body felt like a war zone, constantly threatening me with torture and death. My life was a dance among the mine fields. Any wrong move and I could be blasted from the inside with desperate pain—or killed. I knew and lived terror.

I knew the difficulties of those unable to get around on their own resources. The difficulties of having to rely on elevators—especially when they were out of order, and I had to find many circuitous routes to get to my destination—or where there were none at all, and I simply was denied access. I knew the problems of those without transportation in a city with little mass transit. I had to rely on the schedules and availability and kindheartedness of others. Losing my independence was hard for me, but this is daily reality for the poor, the mentally and physically challenged, the elderly, and the very young.

I learned something of what it is to be old, to be living with a body that doesn't work right anymore, with fears of being especially vulnerable to disease and stroke and attack and the cold and the heat. If I got caught in a fire, if my child were in danger, if I were threatened by an attacker, I couldn't run fast to get away. And I was tired. As I struggled to stay awake at every turn (with Paul pulling on my arm, pleading "Morning, morning," his two-year-old way of saying "Wake up!"), I often wondered if this is what it is to be like to be old, simply needing to lie down with the fatigue of living that accumulates over the years.

And I learned what it was like to be very young. I wanted to be able to care for myself—to make my own meals, wash my own dishes, do my own laundry—and was so frustrated when my well-meaning caretakers wouldn't let me. I was so determined to wash my own hair in the hospital that I set off an episode of tachycardia that nearly killed me. My then eighteen-month-old son was, at the same time, struggling to do whatever he could for and by himself. Every attempt to put food in his mouth, put clothes on his body, climb the stairs, open a door was accompanied by "Me do." I learned to respect his every effort at independence. Paul and I struggled together to gain our autonomy.

In the midst of this search for something good in all of this, I had discovered an empathic perspective. But more than empathy, I had discovered the transformative power of gratitude. The power to make of a curse, a blessing. The power to make of an absence, an abundance. I had learned, once again (for it was not the first time this lesson had been taught to me) that when I focused on what I didn't have, I had a closet full of clothes and nothing to wear, a houseful of books and nothing to read, a life full of opportunity and nothing to do. When I focused on what I did have, the handful of fish and the few loaves of bread became enough to feed a multitude. Thankfulness. An appreciation of what we have at hand. It fills our lives and makes our lives fulfilling.

Yet even with this knowledge and change in perspective, my gratitude at this point was still primarily intellectual, heady. It was a change of perspective, but was it a change of heart? It seems that true gratitude is heartfelt. It cuts deeper. It isn't just an appreciation of the fullness of one's life. It is the fullness itself. When we are grateful we are full—full of gratitude.

The gratitude I'm talking about is that of the father for the prodigal son, the gratitude for that which was lost, that now is found. That amazing grace that fills us when something that we feared lost is returned to us. In our losing it, or nearly losing it, it becomes all the more precious.

My spirit dog companion, Juniper, who shared my life for eleven years, was a wild and free spirit, and I cherished this in her, but it also gave her the propensity to wander off from our walks together in pursuit of some wilder animal or perhaps simply a flight of fancy. Nevertheless, she would often disappear and not return home for hours. Though she always returned, each time I would wonder and worry if this was the time she would not come home, that she would become lost or injured or killed by a speeding car. Each time, I lost her in my heart, and each time when she returned home, I was filled to tears with the preciousness of her. I was so very grateful that she was returned to me.

In his first few weeks of kindergarten and learning the ropes and rules of bus riding and going to and from the bus, my then five-year-old son failed to come home on time. When I learned of this (I was at work), my mind filled with fears of accidents and kidnappings, of my child being gone from me forever. I rushed to my car, needing to find him somehow. As I approached my house, there he was, slowly walking home. He had stopped off to say hello to a neighbor and simply stayed. I got out of the car, held him tight in my arms, and wept. He wondered why I was crying. It was simply the fullness of my gratitude pouring out.

There is a feeling of fullness in gratitude, a feeling that one simply cannot contain it all. It fills one up and spills over . . .

> *Filling up and spilling over, it's an endless waterfall*
> *Filling up and spilling over, over all.*
>
> CRIS WILLIAMSON, "Waterfall"

I think that's often why we weep when full of gratitude. I find I weep a lot lately.

At some point in this journey of my heart, probably some time after my second arrest, this deeper sense of gratitude began to grow in me. As the reality of the tenuousness of my life sank in, I began to see each day as a gift. I lived on the edge of lost and found; every day held the potential of my losing my life, and every day I found life again. This seemed particularly poignant to me each night as I tucked my little boy in his bed, wondering if I would live through the night. As I left his room, I would say, "See you in the morning," more in prayer than in certainty. And I began each day with a "thank you" for living through the night and finding my sweet baby in my arms once more.

This sense of the fragility and preciousness of our time together pervaded our whole family. Thankfulness became a part of our family's daily ritual. Gathering around the table at dinnertime, we would hold hands with one another and say grace, and that grace always included a thank you for one more day of being together.

Grace. Graci. Gracias. Thank you . . . We say grace by giving thanks. And so I came to see the connection between grace and gratitude— grace as gratitude and gratitude as grace. I had often felt uncomfortable with the concept of grace, especially the grace of God, as it is associated in my mind with exclusivity, as something only a select and elect few could attain. But thinking of gratitude as grace and grace as gratitude opened my vision of grace, made me see it as being more than the favor of God. Perhaps grace is God's gratitude for all of creation.

According to the *Oxford English Dictionary*, grace includes the divine influence to regenerate and sanctify and to impart strength to endure trial and resist temptation. I had been seeking a way to regenerate my spirit, to endure the trials of deprivation and resist the temptations of bitterness and resentment. I had turned to gratitude. And I found grace.

I must have had a sense of this connection between gratitude and grace long before I became cognizant of it. In a bittersweet moment prior to my transplant, several months after my first arrest, I wrote:

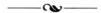

Life—so elusive. I dance on the shores of it and dive into its deep pools. I bounce on its waves and am dragged under by its undertow. I glide across its calm surface. I marvel at its immensity and purity. I want to grasp it all in my arms. It is too large . . . I am baptized by its grace.

DECEMBER 1, 1990

What is it to live in grace? To be gracious? I suppose it is this: to be living in a state of gratitude. In her reflections on gratitude, Joan Borysenko writes of the Jewish custom of praying frequently throughout the day by thanking God for the little things—washing hands, entering a house, seeing the first star at night. It is this ordinary gratitude and gratitude for the ordinary, a daily appreciation of the ever-present gifts of our life that we so easily take for granted, that grants us grace. Living in the fullness of such continuing gratitude, we have little room for greed, or resentment, or hostility. I know that even at my grumpiest, a remembrance of the gifts of my life will quickly restore in me the fullness and joy of gratitude. Of grace.

Sometimes I think the real gift I received in receiving this new heart is not the gift of life itself so much as the gift of knowing gratitude in such a deep and profound way. For it was with my literal change of heart that I became vividly aware that what once had been lost now was found, and I was so deeply grateful. I had the rare opportunity of nearly losing my life, and having it restored in me. But it was more than restored. In the losing and the restoration I found a new and deeper dimension to my life. Perhaps I had in a strange way stumbled across the meaning of Christ's teaching that whoever would find their life must first lose it. I had lost so much of my life, and now it was returned to me, and it seemed sevenfold. In the losing of my life, I had found so much. I had found a fullness, a gratitude, a grace. It took a change of heart to bring out my deepest gratitude. I have known nothing like it.

I can never express the profundity of literally having my life restored to me. Yet, so often the overwhelming sense of gratitude has come with those moments of the tangible return of the small things that had been lost, those "first time" experiences—the first time I returned to my sacred spot and found myself weeping with gratitude all along the path; the first time I was able to hike up into the mountains in the fall; the first winter storm when I could go out and frolic in the snow rather than being concerned that I was cut off from hospitals and ambulances. The first time I was able to perform again with Jody and Mary was especially meaningful to me. I was so scared to be getting up on stage again, afraid that the horror would happen all over again, but when I began to play the music, my heart took over and we entered into it together. When we were finished, again I wept, not in sorrow or even relief, but in deep gratitude that this precious part of my life was restored to me. What was lost had been found.

I am grateful, deeply grateful to my donor and her family. I am grateful, deeply grateful to my husband, and my sister, and my brothers, and my extended family, and my friends, and all those many unnamed others who have given so generously of themselves on my behalf. But my deepest and most profound gratitude is for the ordinariness of life. These are the things I never again want to take for granted. What it is to awake in the morning with no sense of impending doom, anticipating the day. What it is to walk—what an incredible privilege. I cry at every step and become the waterfall. To watch the sunrise. For years I had been too drugged and doped and simply scared to rise with the sun. I had lost the sunrise, and now it was found. Every morning brings blessedness.

———— ❧ ————

*It is so beautiful here I can hardly stand it. It is the early
morning with its pale colors and light. The sun is rising over
the hills as the seagulls fly overhead. It is very calm and still.*

*A doe has come to visit me a couple times in the past week.
I can't help but feeling she is my spirit doe. It is as if she knows
I am recovering my self.*

I am so grateful to be alive, fully alive again.

JUNE 10, 1994

I am so grateful for life and all its accompanying gifts—be they
wonders or woes. Even the most arduous tasks become a challenge, something to be savored. I am glad for them in a way I never knew before.
Just to walk in the woods again, to dance, to dive into a clear cool lake,
to work up a good sweat, to enter into a passionate discussion, to feel a
lightness in my being, to tuck my little boy in at night knowing I'll be
there when he wakes up in the morning. I am so very grateful.

Yet I have found that it is not enough for me to be thankful. I have
a desire to do something in return. To do thanks. To give thanks. Give
things. Give thoughts. Give love. So gratitude becomes the gift, creating a cycle of giving and receiving, the endless waterfall. Filling up and
spilling over. To give from the fullness of my being. This comes not
from a feeling of obligation, like the child's obligatory thank-you notes
to grandmas and aunts and uncles after receiving presents. Rather, it is
a spontaneous charitableness, perhaps not even to the giver but to
someone else, to whoever crosses one's path. It is the simple passing on
of the gift.

I have known a certain frustration in trying to express my gratitude to my donor family. Nothing can repay the deed. All I can do is
to give of my life, to make my life a gift, to be gracious in my living,
which is to live in gratitude and thus grace.

Joy

*"I've got the joy, joy, joy, joy—
down in my heart"*

CAMP SONG

The summer solstice was indeed the longest day of the year for me, not because of the long sunlight, but because of the long wait. That was the day I would find out if the treatment for rejection had been effective. The phone seemed to ring a lot that day, but it never was the call I was waiting for. We went to a lake with some friends, simply to escape the house and the phone and the waiting. Still, I checked the answering machine first thing when we got home. No message.

At last, the call. I was clear. The rejection had stopped. The tears poured out of me, a waterfall of tears at the gladness of the reprieve. I was alive! I wasn't dying now, and I wasn't dying soon. "Grateful" is too small a word to capture the depth of what I was feeling. I was alive I was alive I was alive. I wanted to shout it to the world, so I went to the one place in the world that I have always felt most fully alive—the great sand beach—and there on the night of the summer solstice Sam (my dog) and I ran the length of the beach, reveling in the tail ends of the last rays of the sun on that longest day. The beach stretched before us as the sun stretched out the day as my life now stretched before me in a way that it hadn't until that moment. I was going to live to live to live to love to shout to run to dance about in the waves we ran and ran and ran and ran . . . We sat for a long time on that beach gazing out at the water that found no end in the sky, just as my life no longer saw its end, and we rejoiced! Oh, how we rejoiced! My heart was full, and God's grace was all about me. This sun, this sand, this great clear lake. As we slowly walked back, the moon began to rise, so looking in one direction we saw the setting sun and looking in the other direction we saw the rising moon. We were encircled in the heavens, and I was alive! Yes! I embrace it with such profound joy.

That one day encapsulated the whole experience of the transplant—the long wait, the wondering whether or not I would live, the deep and profound joy at being graced by another chance to embrace this life. This great gift of another chance to live, and to live *well* in all senses of the word, brought such great joy to my heart. I had the joy, joy, joy, joy, down in my heart. The song says it all. Joy, joy, joy, joy. Saying it once simply isn't enough. It begs to be repeated. Joy, joy, joy, joy!—and it is down—down deep. Joy is a deep wellspring, its source deep below the surface, unaffected by the surface conditions—the winds of change, the cracks in the earth's crust—a constant source, never running dry, and then bubbling up, an effervescence, and overflowing, constantly renewing. The joy bubbled out of me. I wanted to embrace everyone and everything. I simply could not contain it.

In those first late spring days after the transplant, every moment tapped into that wellspring and brought forth joy. The sunrise, the seagulls flying through the mists, early morning birdsongs, standing without fear in the shower and feeling each drop of warm water soak my skin, the sun strong upon my back, my body weary with use, the rain upon my face, the splashing of waves on my feet, running up the stairs to get the phone, the brightly lit faces of old friends as they first set eyes upon me as though I had returned from the dead—all of them moments for joy.

Such a joy, simply to be alive! In the years before my transplant, I had so longed for life . . .

———— ❧ ————

On mornings like this, when the spring sunshine comes streaming in, I awake almost happy. There's something in the angle and the color of the light this time of year that is so hopeful. I can almost feel the world coming back to life.

I can feel it in me, and perhaps that's why the thought of dying is especially poignant right now. I am so filled with life. I want to embrace it. And I fear that it will be snatched away from me. I need time; I want time. Time to love my baby boy and watch him grow. Time with my sweet David. Time to plant trees and flowers and watch them blossom. Time to pull together the knowledge and the wisdom I've accumulated in this lifetime and pass it on. Time to give of myself what I can to make others' lives better. Time to walk by the lake and hike in the hills and paddle a canoe.

I hear people complain about the big and little problems in their lives and I want to say "You're alive. You're well. Rejoice!" What a gift this life is.

MARCH 12, 1992

. . . and here it was given to me.

Yet I learned to be cautious in my joyousness. Though I was treated successfully for the rejection, for awhile after that initial burst of joy on the solstice, I was afraid to feel the joy, fearing somehow that I would be punished for being so joyous, as if I were allowed only so much happiness in a lifetime and no more. But joy is irrepressible. Perhaps one can cap it for a time, keep it bottled up, but eventually it will burst forth again. For me, every change of season after the transplant tapped into the wellspring of joy.

Spring. I first began to walk again in the springtime. What a sweet delight to be out in the breeze, to hear the birdsong, to be among the other revelers of spring. Sometimes the steps were painful. I didn't have the stamina to go far. But it didn't matter, I was so glad to be a part of it again. And to walk without fear.

Summer. Early in the summer, we took Paul on his first camping trip. To be in the woods, far from home, far from help, and be unafraid—oh this was a deep and grateful joy.

It had been so many years since I had woken up in the woods, seen the early morning mists on the lake, heard the call of the loon. To share it all with Paul, finally—to watch him discover the delights of cooking over a fire, paddling in the canoe, tromping around in the muck at the water's edge, sitting by the fire late at night, cuddling up cozily in the tent—doubled the joy.

Summer also brought the joy of running barefoot on the beach. No matter how old I am, I always feel myself youthful, lithe, light—free—as my toes play tag with the waves as we chase each other up and down the beach. I am so fully alive there.

And at last to plunge myself with total abandon into the water itself.

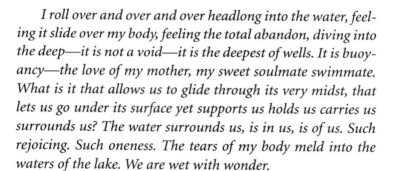

I roll over and over and over headlong into the water, feeling it slide over my body, feeling the total abandon, diving into the deep—it is not a void—it is the deepest of wells. It is buoyancy—the love of my mother, my sweet soulmate swimmate. What is it that allows us to glide through its very midst, that lets us go under its surface yet supports us holds us carries us surrounds us? The water surrounds us, is in us, is of us. Such rejoicing. Such oneness. The tears of my body meld into the waters of the lake. We are wet with wonder.

JULY 1994

Abandon. Oneness. This is joy.

Fall. The colors so bright, the air so crisp and clear—the hills beckoned. Finally I could be up in them, moving my body up against the weight of the hill—far, far up until we were at the top of the world overlooking this bright blue lake and sky and crimson and gold hills—

a celebration of color in every direction. I wept with gratitude and rejoicing, so glad I was to be a part of it again.

Winter. The winters of the previous years had been hard. Each big snowstorm meant being trapped, cut off from emergency medical support. But not this year. The first big snow of the season fell with such delight in my heart and with such bluster. The snow began at dusk, and soon Paul and I were out in the dark, standing in the swirling snows, barely able to see each other, so strong were the snows and winds. We reveled in it. We frolicked and romped and slid down the hill. I stood for a long time with the snow pelting my upturned face. It was winter! It was snowing! And I was alive, fully alive! With arms outstretched and face to the heavens, I embraced it with such joy.

I had gone through the dark night of my life, and in this new morning of my life, I knew such joy.

"Weeping may tarry for the night,
but joy comes with the morning."

PSALM 30:5

Early morning has a certain quality not unlike the quality of this new life that lay ahead of me, a creative solitude before the noise and busyness of the day. Only the few are awake. The birds sound different. The air smells different—fresher. We feel a sense of possibility. Dawn. A new day dawning. The dawning of new possibilities. And a splendor in the sunrise.

In the years of my illness, I had missed the mornings and their accompanying joy. The drugs left me dopey. I could not rouse myself for the sunrise, and when I did awake, joy escaped me. Often in my life, I would awaken from a bad dream with a feeling of relief and joy upon discovering that it was only a dream. During these years of illness, I often experienced the reverse. I would dream of life as it had been—happy, healthy, free—only to awake to the bad dream I lived. Each morning, I awoke to that same sense of doom and dread. Something is wrong. Something is really wrong. What is it? Then I would feel the bulge in my stomach, feel my heart, and remember, oh yes. It is this nightmare. Perhaps the worst of all of this was to awaken without joy, without a sense of possibility in the day. My mother always told me that joy comes with the morning, but it didn't. The weeping often tarried through the night and far into the day.

But I could not live all day, each day, in the doom and gloom. I needed, as Albert Camus has said,

> *in order to prevent [myself] . . .*
> *from shriveling up, from becoming nothing but a*
> *magnificent orange with a dry, bitter pulp, . . .*
> *[to] keep a freshness and a source of joy intact within . . .*
>
> *. . . In the worst years of our madness the memory of this sky*
> *had never left me. It was this that in the end had saved me*
> *from despair. . . .*
>
> *In Tipasa, the world is born again each day in a light always*
> *new. . . .*
>
> *In the depths of winter, I finally learned that within me*
> *lay an invincible summer.*
>
> ALBERT CAMUS, *Return to Tipasa*

In order to prevent my heart from shriveling up, in order to keep myself from becoming dry and bitter, I needed to keep a source of joy intact. I needed a Tipasa, an invincible summer.

My traditional sources of joy—the sunrise, being out in the woods, dancing, swimming with abandon, a fearless solitude that gave my soul time and space to renew—were closed to me. But as surely as I would rise with a sense of doom and gloom, so surely would my son rise soon after and walk into my room with a smile and a "good morning," so delighted for the day that I thought, yes, it must be a good morning after all. What a continual source of delight he was to me in all of this. He was my source of joy, and he kept me intact, even in the worst years.

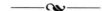

Christmas has come and gone. You have filled it with such delight for all of us.

When I read to you at night, I see the sparkle of Christmas tree lights reflected in your eyes. For all of us, Christmas has been seen through your eyes.

It has been such fun to decorate the tree with you and cut out Christmas cookies and hear you sing "Frosty the Snowman" and " Jingle Bells" and "Deck the Halls" over and over again.

And you are so giving and generous and so inwardly and outwardly joyous. You seem to be the spirit of Christmas itself.

Thank you for all you bring to our lives, sweet one. You are the greatest joy and the deepest love I have ever known.

TO PAUL, DECEMBER 30, 1991

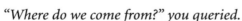

Living with you is such a delight. Everything is a source of excitement to you. I think the Latin root of "enthusiasm" must have meant "three-year-old." Last night when you were taking your bath you cried out excitedly, "Look, they [your hands] don't clap under water!" Every little thing is a wonderful discovery.

TO PAUL, MARCH 12, 1992

"Where do we come from?" you queried.

We gave you a variety of biological, spiritual, and evolutionary answers, and then you said, "I think we come from butterflies."

TO PAUL, AUGUST 27, 1992

Paul was my source of joy. No matter how despondent I was, the sight of that smiling face, and he does have a quick and ready smile, beaming upon mine brought joy and life to me. Perhaps it was the contagion of his own spirit. Young children seem possessed of an irrepressible joy—the freshness of life, the delight of discovery, the sense of possibility, the gift of life lived in the moment.

I believe we are all born with this capacity for joy. Certain things tap into it—a Bach sonata, a Bob Marley song, the first rays of the sun, the flashing color of the goldfinch, the hand of a child placed trustfully in yours; others cap it—pain, social expectations, various imprisonments of the body and soul. My longing, in those years of waiting, to be alive, fully alive, was not simply a longing to extend the years of my life—the defibrillator purportedly was doing that—but to be ALIVE with the joy I knew myself capable of.

I want to feel full of life again. I want to live without preoccupation, without hesitation. I want to live wholeheartedly. . . .

I want to love this life with abandon, to give expression to the "yes!"

JULY 28 and NOVEMBER 5, 1992

To live and love wholeheartedly, without hesitation, with total abandon, is to be open to that joy which is the wellspring of our being. The gift of a new heart is a gift of life indeed. Now, with my healthy and whole heart, I could open to the joy.

I've come full circle now, back through spring and on into summer. Still, each season renews the blessing.

Now I sit on my summer hill, a quiet joy gladdening my heart. It is my second season here—the joy not so intense, but present nonetheless. It is such a joy to be here, to embrace the day without fear, to live it in gladness and with true knowledge of the gift of it all.

JULY 1995

Celebration

———— ❧ ————

*All the colors of hope and joy and celebration swirl around
me today.*

*Oh, Dick and Tony, your balloons have reminded me that
we are celebrating—I hear the joy from all corners.*

I listen to my music, I hear the voices

Barb had her baby—new life—new soul—

Oh the circle of people

Thank you for this privilege

*I wish I could gather all these people around me. I feel that
they are all here.*

MARCH 2, 1994

My first few days following my transplant operation were
spent in a stupor at best, in drugged hallucinations of
dragons and demons at worst. I was vaguely aware of the
cards and calls and well wishes that had been pouring in, but I was not
fully awake to the gathering celebration.

Shortly after my transplant, there arrived in my room a great bouquet of red, yellow, and blue balloons, which lifted my spirit and
brought it into the atmosphere of celebration that had been swirling
round my fringes all these days. Listening to my tape of "spirit songs,"

I let myself be embraced by the music and the color and the great gladness.

> *"Love of my life," I am crying, I am not dying,*
> *I am dancing,*
> *Dancing along in the madness, there is no sadness,*
> *Only a song of the soul.*
> *And we'll sing this song, why don't you sing along*
> *And we can sing for a long, long time.*
> *. . . And we can sing for a long, long time.*
>
> CRIS WILLIAMSON, "Song of the Soul"

The sounds and sights tossed me up in the air; carried me on their shoulders; danced me around the room. YES! It is done and it is good. This is cause for celebration. Bring out the balloons, ring the bells, shout it from the mountaintops, dance it down the streets. I am not dying. I am dancing. Life is good. It is time for CELEBRATION!

And it was if they all were with me—friends, family, strangers in the street—all dancing, singing, joining hands and hearts and hopes. Such a circle dance. "Love has drawn a circle," sings Kate Wolf. The circle reached out, welcoming each, all joined together in this jubilation.

Love has drawn a circle . . . cards and phone calls poured in from all around the country and beyond. The cards were not ordinary "get well" cards, or even "wishing you well on your recovery from your operation" cards. They were cards of congratulations and celebration. So many came with the message that they all were celebrating.

> When I first heard the news of your surgery, my emotions soared—elation and fear simultaneously. For the first week, I could hardly think of anything else—so hoping that your recovery would proceed well. Now that all the news has been positive, the elation is all that remains. I am so very happy for you! Somehow a "get well" card is too ordinary; . . . You are most certainly to be congratulated. . . . You did it!

> Jody called and gave me the news. . . . I couldn't believe my

ears! I was so very, very happy. I can't even speak of how happy I am—for me, for you, for your family—and for the world at large. . . . Your spirit will triumph.

I only heard the good news today. I felt like jumping up and down. It is most wonderful.

"Congratulations!"

"I am so happy!"

I am in awe . . . more than the birth process (from a friend who had been with me at Paul's birth).

Yes—yes—YES! I heard the news (we've been waiting for soooo long.) Congratulations with your new heart (goose bumps all over just hearing about it). I am so very, very, very happy for you, Beth!

YEAH, BETH!

The circle widened. At the university, the secretary in our department kept all members of the campus community regularly informed on my progress. I heard from students, faculty, staff across campus. They all seemed to be rejoicing.

At our church, our minister hung a huge banner in the office window, "BETH GOT HER HEART!" announcing the good news to all who came through there. A few days before my transplant, a friend and valued and respected member of our community died. Her memorial service was held at our church the day after my transplant. All who came to celebrate Fran's life also passed the banner with the good news. Mutual friends of ours later told me how good it was to be able to celebrate a "new" life along with the passing of Fran's.

A few days after my transplant, Mary and Jody were once again giving a concert at the coffeehouse where I had first arrested. They began with the announcement that I had received my new heart. "Everyone clapped and cheered and whistled . . . " (from a note written by a friend). I felt as though I could hear it a hundred miles away, so much did I feel the uplifting of so many spirits.

And the circle widened more. I got cards and messages from people I wouldn't have expected to know about the transplant, sometimes from people I hardly knew. How eagerly people spread good news. Just a few days after my transplant, I heard from a friend from high school who lives near my hometown, a thousand miles away.

> I heard this morning that you are the proud "owner" of a new heart! I'm so very happy for you! My mother heard it from Mrs. Loughridge, Karyn's mom, who heard it from Karyn, who learned it from Mrs. Baird, who is in a wellness class she teaches. . . . How's that for a "good news" network!

Perhaps my case was unusual in that so much of my struggle had been so public—both my arrests had been witnessed by hundreds of people, had touched hundreds of lives—but I was so struck by the ever-widening community of people who were drawn into the circle of celebration. Even more than this, I was struck by the genuineness of their rejoicing. It was as if they had been with me through it all; as if we had gone through arduous rapids and over the falls together—and then emerged jubilant and triumphant in the calm, smooth waters. This was not my private joy. So many were celebrants with me.

I had discovered the element of compassion inherent in celebration. I have always thought of compassion as a sharing of sufferings, and surely, given the depth of their rejoicing, all of these people must have suffered with me as well. But here I discovered that compassion is not only a matter of suffering with, but also rejoicing with. They rejoiced in my rejoicing; my joys were their joys.

"To rejoice at another person's joy is like being in heaven," says Meister Eckhart.

How often do we truly rejoice at another's joys? It seems that so often we see others' good fortune coming at our expense, as though we are competing for power, honor, glory, and there's only so much to go around. Our celebrations—our compassionate rejoicing—are tempered by resentment, competition. I struggled with that for years whenever a friend was pregnant. It was so hard to be glad for them. Certainly it's not that there are only so many babies to go around.

Their good fortune did nothing to deprive me. But it pained me nevertheless. Their good fortune seemed like an arrow aimed at my heart, just another jab pointing out my deprivation, a mocking of my loss. Being so centered on my own griefs, losses, and deprivations blocked the impulse toward genuine celebration.

We learn early on to pick a team and root for our side—to rejoice in our victories and their defeats. Celebration calls on us to root for everyone. In one of her Christmas letters, Dave's cousin described the swimming races at Courage Center, where everyone encourages everyone else, and the one who comes in last gets the biggest cheer of all simply for making it. She remarked at what a wonderful world it would be if the rest of life was like that.

That's what I awoke to on that day, the day the balloons arrived in my hospital room, the day the whole world was cheering me on. How great if we could all do that for each other and know that it comes not at our expense, at our deprivation. Another's victories do not diminish us, deprive us. Rather, others' good fortune only enhances our own.

> *We must rejoice in their joys as much as in our own joys,*
> *we must long for their honor as much as for our own honor,*
> *and we must love a stranger as our own relatives.*
> *In this way, people are constantly in joy and honor,*
> *and a good situation, just as if they were in the kingdom of*
> *heaven. Thus they have more frequent joys*
> *than if they only had a joy in their own benefits.*
>
> MEISTER ECKHART, *Sermons*

This is the true spirit of celebration to which I awoke on that day. I had never known the fullness of others' compassion—of others loving me as they love themselves—until that moment, with the full openhearted rejoicing of others with me. To celebrate is to rejoice with, for ultimately, celebration is, as Eckhart says, about loving others as we love ourselves. Sharing in their sufferings, rejoicing in their joys.

Celebration. *Kagiyaah* in Hebrew, which comes from the word "kag," meaning to draw a circle around. "Love has drawn a circle."

Celebration is love drawing a circle. I felt encircled by love, celebration, and rejoicing. It was a circle dance.

The circle widened further. The balloons gave a spirit of celebration to everyone entering the room. Nurses would come in just to spend a few moments in this spirit of celebration. Certainly most of their work there must be filled with the hardship and messiness of life. Here they could take a few moments to celebrate. Even strangers passing by on their way to other rooms would come in and pause a moment to lift up their spirits before passing on down the hall.

Here in the hospital and in the messages of joy and jubilation I received from the world beyond, I felt people's deep and genuine need to celebrate. To celebrate is to say YES. This is good. Celebration is affirmation. We need celebrations to renew and sustain our spirits.

I don't think that I ever fully appreciated the need to celebrate until that day. So many of our celebrations—of birthdays, graduations, Christmas —have become more frenzied than festive, more expected than expectant, more an outpouring of money than of joy— that in the busyness of our daily lives they are more an encumbrance than a delight. I think of the times of great fatigue prior to the transplant, when I simply didn't have the energy to celebrate Paul's birthday or cook a Thanksgiving dinner. I didn't realize then how the celebration could feed me.

Perhaps the darkest times are when we most need to celebrate. Indeed, celebrations are the triumphant emergence out of darkness. Rarely do I feel the spirit of celebration so strongly as I do on the night of the winter solstice. There is always a feeling that we have made it. We as a people, especially up here in the North where our winter darkness is so much a part of the day, have made it to the point of the greatest darkness, and now each day will bring more light. Such a feeling of celebration there is on that longest night of the year. In the past several years, I have joined in a solstice celebration with others. We form the circle, remembering the year past, and honoring the qualities and the people that have brought us through the year, then leap over the fire in anticipation of the new year.

It seems that the spirit of celebration necessarily includes the leaping over the fire—the overcoming of trials and sorrows, the testings of our spirit. Celebration is triumphant—over death, struggle, over forces of darkness. We celebrate our victories, be they large or small.

We have so many occasions for celebration. We tend to think of celebrations as gala occasions—a golden wedding anniversary, a college graduation, the birth of a baby—but every day presents occasions for celebration. The small triumphs of life—the idea bursting forth, the sunrise, an unexpected rainbow, the first crocuses in the spring, the first snowflakes in November, learning how to tie shoes, finally getting the pie crust right . . .

One of the great delights of the first year of a baby's life is that it seems an endless celebration—the first smile, the first rolling over, the first attempts at crawling, the first tooth, the first steps—all occasions for great glee and celebration. So is the first year of life after a transplant—the first walk, the first stairs, the first time alone in the woods, the first venturing far from home, the first swim . . .

What I had most missed about the summer was being able to swim. Oh, I had been able to dip my body in the water—but not swim. Not dive under the water in celebration and sensuality. My first swim. It was like being baptized. To dive into the water unafraid. There is no greater abandon. Merging with my mother—she held me—and Juniper was there beside me too and we swam, our spirits swimming together—we are all one—the water, the spirit, and they on the dock—all of them laughing in the delight of my delight, rejoicing with me, ah the celebration of life . . .
JULY 1994

The first dance . . .

Today I danced. I thought my dancing days were over—I might as well have given up my soul. But today, today, with

Paul's hands in mine and the music in my heart I danced. We danced—Paul, myself, all of the others—the children, the grown, all in a circle of life. I feel the lightness—my spirit soars—my body heart and soul joining with the rhythms. I become one with the music—with the others dancing we become a great circle of celebration—the whirling twirling celebration of life. Hands joined to hands—the rejoicing spreads from one to another like electricity through our bodies, joined at our very core. The circle takes us to the very center of the great gleeful gladness.

SEPTEMBER 1994

All the firsts. All the small triumphs. The trick is to keep that spirit of celebration alive, not let it get sucked up in the necessities of daily life. Yet celebration is itself a necessity of life. It is itself sustaining—a sustenance of the human spirit.

Make a joyful noise . . . the Psalms say over and over again.

Make a joyful noise to the Lord, all the earth;
break forth into joyous song and sing praises!
Sing praises to the Lord with the lyre,
with the lyre and the sound of melody!
With trumpets and the sound of the horn
make a joyful noise before the King, the Lord!
Let the sea roar, and all that fills it;
the world and those who dwell in it!
Let the floods clap their hands;
let the hills sing for joy together

PSALM 98:4–8

We need to celebrate. It is good to affirm our existence, our together being, our triumphs large or small. And we need to share our celebrations. Our celebrations ring hollow in isolation. We want to embrace and be embraced in our good news.

The spirit of celebration calls us to honor the moment. I think of Paul celebrating the loss of his first tooth. He was so anxious in the hours before, when the tooth began to wiggle. It was a trial. Would it hurt? Would he swallow it? And then, in a moment, it was out. YES! YES! YES! he shouted, running up and down the street, calling forth his joy. And it wasn't enough that he experience this triumph himself. He ran to tell Lynn and his friends; he called his favorite aunts when he got home; he recounted the story at kindergarten the next day and had his name placed in the ranks of "lost tooth club." This was something to celebrate, something to rejoice in and commemorate in a communal way.

So much of life gives us cause to celebrate, especially when our circle widens beyond our personal joys and triumphs to include those of others.

My transplant and the ensuing celebration reminded me that we are a jubilant, triumphant, celebrant, and compassionate people. Our spirits do rise up; every day presents opportunities for celebration. Our celebrations don't have to be elaborate galas, planned down to every detail. The true celebration comes in these spontaneous outpourings of our heart. We simply need to allow them room.

To celebrate is to honor, to commemorate. Celebration calls on us to honor the moment. Honor it with spontaneous celebration. With singing and dancing, with lyre and trumpet and exultation. At times, in the midst of the struggle, pausing to celebrate can feel so indulgent, almost inappropriate. But it is the very stuff of life. There is "a time to mourn, and a time to dance" (Ecclesiastes 3:4). Celebration is the affirmation that we are here and life, at this moment, is good. If we can't celebrate that, what's the point of the rest? As Emma Goldman said, "If I can't dance, I don't want to be part of the revolution." Times of mourning will come again; we will grieve; but for the moment, we can dance and rejoice.

For years, our mother had told us that she wanted Rodgers and Hammerstein's "Shall We Dance?" played at her memorial service— and we did. I suppose that people might have thought it odd, but I remember doing it with such great glee. Now it strikes me as the most appropriate of songs—an invitation to join in the great cosmic celebration.

To celebrate is to honor each other. When we celebrate, we wish each other well. The spirit of celebration calls on us all to join the circle—and dance.

Guilt, grief, and forgiveness

And you're flowing like a river,
the changer and the changed.

CRIS WILLIAMSON

My celebrations were tempered by guilt. At first it was guilt simply at being so joyous, so celebrative, when somebody somewhere was grieving the loss of their child, the very child whose heart brought such celebration to my life. Each bit of celebration—my first outing to the zoo, my first homecoming, my first hike in the woods, my first run down the sledding hill—was shrouded on the edges by guilt. Here I was out enjoying life and doing all the things a kid would be doing. She should be out doing them, not me. She should have this chance; I've had mine. She never got hers.

I felt guilt for profiting from the death of another. Like a thief plundering the bodies of the dead on a battlefield, I had plundered this body, but for something far more valuable than watches and wallets. I had plundered her for her very heart itself. It is a strange and difficult thing about transplantation, that one's life comes so directly at the expense of another. Waiting for a new heart, circling like a vulture for someone else to die is hard enough. In the actual receiving, in carrying the very heart of another inside oneself, one feels the sense of pillage so intensely.

The guilt for being happy in the midst of their grief grew to a guilt for being alive. The question I hear asked by so many transplant recipients is "Why me?" meaning not "Why did this awful thing happen to me that I should need a transplant?" but rather "Why am I so lucky? Why am I still alive, and they are dead? Why me? Why me?"

I thought for a long time that I certainly could never look my donor's family in the eye, so deep was my guilt at being alive while their daughter had died. How must her family feel that I can go on and do all these things that she will never have the chance to do?

The guilt grew larger. Not only did I feel guilt for being alive at the cost of J.'s life, the guilt grew to a generalized guilt for being alive while anyone died, especially the young.

About the time of my transplant, a friend of a friend, who was about my age and had a young child, died of a sudden acute illness. Even though I did not know him, hearing of his death, knowing the depth of my friend's loss, I felt such guilt for being alive. It was supposed to be me—not him.

About the same time, the nineteen-year-old son of an acquaintance was murdered. Again, the waves of guilt flooded over me as if I had been the one to pull the trigger. It was supposed to be me—not him.

Then the woman who had taken my place when I was unable to teach, who had received awards for her gifts as a teacher, lost her chance for a permanent teaching job. Far better that I had died and she could have had the place left vacant in my absence.

Later in the summer, a woman about my age, much loved at the university, died in a motorcycle accident. Again, the guilt. So much better had it been me, not her.

A few months after my transplant, I heard on the radio of the death of a much beloved college president, a wonderful teacher, a highly respected and valued member of the community. He had died while waiting for a heart. Why him, not me? So much better had it been me, not him, who died.

I suppose it is something akin to the guilt that some survivors of mass tragedies, of concentration camps, of lost battles feel—the guilt at their own survival, when all around them lie their families and friends and fallen comrades. So did I, with all these worthier people losing their lives all around me, feel guilt at my own survival. I knew my good fortune had not brought their deaths. I knew I had not caused J.'s death. Yet the fact that I held her heart, and rejoiced in it, made me feel somehow responsible. And had I not taken that heart, perhaps someone more worthy than I would have received it. The guilt was becoming unbearable.

There is appropriate guilt, recognizing one's responsibility for harm to others. It is a step towards self-awareness and accountability that can help one to move on. And there is inappropriate guilt—feeling oneself to be bad, wrong, stupid, ashamed for harms for which one is not responsible. And since one is not responsible there is no way of moving out of it. Guilt like the kind I was wallowing in feels like dried up old pudding, paste, glue. It sticks to your ribs, your bones, your skin inside and out. It just sits there, a lump in your stomach—lumpy, gooey, stagnant. It starts to stink. It is hazardous to your health.

It needs to be flushed out. Get that water moving through it.

Mine came out in tears.

It was strange to write J.'s family and tell them all the wonderful things that their gift of J.'s heart had enabled in my life. Their daughter had no chances left, and her heart gave all mine back to me. She was snatched from their arms too soon; her heart let me hold my son a while longer.

Yet it was my correspondence with J.'s family that helped loosen the hold of guilt upon me. In part, the guilt was lessened by their sincere gladness that I could benefit from their loss, and by my, in some way, allowing their daughter to live on. But mostly the guilt was flushed out in an unexpected way.

The more I came to know about J., the more I grieved her loss. I felt a grief for her family's grief, but that was more an empathy for their grief than a grieving in my own soul. There was another grief, a grief that ripped through the center of my being. Yet even this did not feel like my own. Indeed, this felt like J.'s grief. I felt I could sense her not wanting to die. It was as if I could hear her crying out inside my body. For months I lived in a well of deep grief that spilled over and over. It seemed everything made me cry, but especially the thought of that sweet child and her family. I could not talk about her without crying. I cried a river of tears for J. and for her family.

Some transplant centers are reluctant for there to be too much contact between recipients and donor families. They are reluctant for the recipient to know too much about the donor, and vice versa. Part of that is out of respect for the privacy of all parties involved, but I imagine they also know the intense guilt and grief that can accompany the closeness.

When I first felt the waves of grief coming over me, I thought perhaps I knew too much. This was not healthy. The grief was too great. I should not have come so close. But now I see that I needed to take on the grief in order to get through it. The waters of my grief had a cleansing effect, for as the grieving eased, so did the guilt. I needed to know something of J. so that I could take on her pain.

In guilt, one wallows in one's own pain. The grief that healed me was a compassionate grief, feeling the pain of another. Compassion— to suffer with another. I have always appreciated Eleanora Patterson's definition of compassion, that it must include both the choice to suffer with another—as opposed to being flung by fate and circumstance into a situation of suffering; and a sense of self-worth—rather than taking on another's suffering out of a sense of unworth and self-punishment. I did make the choice to know more of J. and her family, and as I did so, my sense of guilt and unworthiness dissipated into a purer grief and compassion. Knowing something of J.'s life, and feeling the attendant compassionate grief, enabled me to move through the guilt. Guilt is self-indulgent and sticky. Grief is a flowing, allowing one to move on.

As Cris Williamson sings, "And you're flowing like a river, the changer, and the changed."

The grief did flow through me, and changed me, enabling me to flow, but there was another element as well. At some point in all this I found forgiveness. The grief was so deep, it seemed it must extend beyond my grieving the loss of this child. Perhaps this grieving was more than that of this child of my heart. Perhaps it was also the grieving of my child self, the one I had blamed all these years for bringing harm to my mother by my birth. Perhaps it was a grieving for all the harms I had ever inflicted. When I had been sick at heart, I felt such a sense of blame, guilt, wrongdoing for which I was being punished. After the transplant, I felt guilt for being alive. But I was not given a new heart simply to wallow in a feeling of "I don't deserve this." That would indeed have been a waste of this gift, a plundering, a slaughter. I had a new heart. Now it was time to forgive—myself. My opening to the possibility of a transplant was a huge step towards forgiveness on my part. I forgave myself enough to give myself another chance. But this was not enough. "Cast away from you all the transgressions which you have committed against me, and get yourselves a new heart and a new spirit!" says Ezekiel. A new heart, *and* a new spirit. It was not enough to get a new heart. Also did I need a new spirit, a spirit of forgiveness. "Cast away from you all the transgressions which you have committed against me"—cast away the transgressions. Let them go. Let go of the guilt. Live. Thrive. Be glad. Rejoice. This is good.

Philosopher Hannah Arendt speaks of forgiveness as being an act of freedom. In forgiving ourselves and others, we *act* rather than *react*. We release ourselves and others from past actions. We do not respond in the expected way. We strike out in a radically new and releasing and freeing direction. We can begin anew. The transplant enabled a new beginning to my life. Only forgiveness allowed me to begin anew.

Every day we are called upon to forgive. "Forgive us our trespasses, as we forgive those who trespass against us." Every day we trespass; every day we are trespassed upon. Forgiveness releases us from the bonds of grudges, resentments, and blame that tie us up, bind up our spirit, prevent our flow, create a self-indulgent guilt. Stuck in that guilt there is nothing to give, no place to go. Forgiveness allows us to flow— to change and be changed.

I think of J. now with a smile. I know the best way I can honor her is not to wallow in guilt, but to go on, cleansed and healed by the grief and the forgiveness.

My celebrations will always have a poignancy now, but far from a destructive guilt that inhibits the spontaneous joy of my spirit, it is more a reverencing of the gift. Reverence, a recognition of the cost of the gifts we receive, is necessary for the sustenance of the spirit and of life. In the spiritual traditions of most Native American hunting tribes, the hunters thank the buffalo or the deer or the rabbit for the gift of its life. In a somewhat similar fashion, our family sometimes practices the Buddhist exercise of mindfulness at a meal, tracing back the origins of the food we have before us. Following the origins of just a can of tomato soup is quite an amazing journey. There is the tomato, which is planted, fertilized, watered, harvested, all with precious resources of people and material. The tomato is then transported, using fossil fuels, in a truck, made of metals and rubber and oil from deep within the earth, which were mined with labor and machines, also made of metals and rubber and oil from deep within the earth. The tomato is processed and placed in a can, also made from metals, and wrapped in paper, from trees that also needed to be grown and harvested and transported. The mindfulness reminds us of the true cost of the gifts we receive. Not that we should feel guilty, but rather that in being so reminded we are less likely to waste or squander these gifts; we are more likely to use them well.

So it is that as I go through my celebrations, and my life, with a reverencing, I am less likely to squander this gift in guilt, but rather to use it well.

Horror and comfort

I will fold you in my arms like a white winged dove
Shine in your soul, your spirit is crying.

CRIS WILLIAMSON

I thought the horror was behind me. In the months after the transplant, I had an occasional flashback. I might awake with a start, certain that I had just been shocked. Or I felt a shock out of the blue in the middle of the day, and then it would be gone. Sometimes I thought that my heart was racing, that I had slipped into tachycardia again. But the flashes were brief. I could put my hands on that space where my defibrillator once resided and assure myself that the dreaded shocking device was gone. I could place my fingers on my pulse and feel it steady, sure. I could rest.

The horror was gone, or so I thought . . .

————— ❧ —————

Last night I entered the horror as I have never done before. We'd been watching Backdraft, *and came to the part in the movie where the badly injured brother is slipping away, his heart beating irregularly. The paramedics call for "lidocaine, now!" Perhaps it was the reminder of the feeling of slipping away, perhaps it was the memory of an urgent demand for lidocaine, but something plunged me back to a moment held*

149

only in the memory of my subconscious—collapsing at Ordean—"I'm going now"—"Lidocaine, more lidocaine"— the incessant shocking—the horror of it all.

The horror of it all. The horror came rushing out at me like the fires that burst out in the backdraft, merely smoldering until that one gasp of oxygen ignites them, creating a fireball of energy. So did my horror, held smoldering for years, explode through my being.

I sobbed uncontrollably for some time, my body and soul heaving. Fearing for my sanity, I cried to David to hold me. I felt myself slipping away, but this time off a cliff of coherence. I got up and walked, hoping to find solace and sanity in a differ-ent place, in the movement itself. But everywhere I turned I knew only the memory of terror. I had been shocked here, and here, and here—at this corner, on this couch, in this bed. I felt entrapped in terror.

Then came the shakes, the trembling, the teeth chattering. I knew I would be okay. That was always my body's signal of relaxation after tachycardia.

I settled in to soothe my heart and mind with videos of Paul as a baby, and a cup of hot chocolate with mounds of whipped cream, and drifted off to sleep.

In the morning I felt like I'd been leached from the in-side—still quite vulnerable, fragile. But the tears didn't come until I got in the shower. There's something about the water that unleashes my own. In the wetness I am freed to weep and wail.

Again fearing for my sanity, I clamored for comfort. It came as I instinctively rocked myself (returning to that moment of rebirthing) and told myself I would be okay. I was soothed, and the soothing came from a maternal presence—the spirit of my mother—the spirit of God. Are they one and the same?

I found myself singing a Christmas carol—"We will rock you, rock you, rock you. We will rock you, rock you, rock you. We will comfort all we can, darling, darling, little lamb." ["Little lamb" was my mother's term of endearment for me, and this was my version of the song; I later found the words to be somewhat different.].

And so I came to Christmas—a story of the hopes and horrors of being born and of being held in the comfort of mother love.

DECEMBER 4, 1994

The impact of that night was manifold. The horror shook my soul to its very core, and I felt weak and vulnerable for several weeks after. I had stored up so much sheer terror inside my soul in all those years in which I could find no safe outlet for all the pain and horror that was coming in, and this wrenching had opened enough of a crack that little bits of horror kept leaking out in surprising ways. Moments of panic. Moments of paranoia. A general feeling of weakness. A wondering if I would ever be whole again. Gradually, it eased.

The other, more profound experience, is with me still. As shaken as I was by the horror, I was even more deeply moved by the comforting presence that enveloped me, calmed my shakes and trembles, warmed my fears. Like my cat, who simply appears every time she hears my son cry, the motherspirit appeared to me, as if in response to my cries. The spirit mother heard my cries, folded me in her arms, rocked me, sang me a lullaby. The presence was so unexpected and yet so comforting. I have felt it before, this deep, deep comfort of a spirit of mother love—a soothing presence gracing my life. Always it has come upon me softly, sometimes as a holding, sometimes as a touch upon the cheek, sometimes as a light kiss upon the forehead. Always with a presence of comfort. A comfort, and a mystery.

And the mystery continued to unfold. The next morning, as I sat in my minister's office, trying to pull together all the fragments of thoughts, inspiration, and my self that were crashing about after my fall, somewhere in that midst was again the presence and the knowledge of comfort. Something I read, or something my minister said, spoke of the Holy Spirit as the Comforter. Perhaps I had come across this before at another time in my life, but it struck me with such

151

vividness now. The Holy Spirit, the Comforter, the Mother—of course. I had known for some time that the Hebrew word for spirit, *ruah*, had feminine connotations, and I had for some time thought of the Holy Spirit as feminine, but never had I particularly associated it with comfort. I had thought of the spirit as power, love, wisdom, strength, grace, protection even, but not comfort, yet that was the powerful feeling holding me now. The spirit of my mother—the spirit of God—are they one and the same? Yes, the Holy Spirit, the Comforter, the Great Mother Goddess. All one and the same.

The mystery unfolded more as I picked up a book (one of those other mysteries—a book simply presents itself, and it is exactly what I need to read) and there it was, Jean Shinoda Bolen talking about the Great Mother Goddess as the Comforter, and then of the Holy Spirit, descending in the form of a dove, a feminine symbol, called the Comforter.

I was captivated by this discovery. God as Mother, as Comforter. Of course. Yes. This resonated in my being. According to Jean Shinoda Bolen, it was right in the New Testament. I needed to read it for myself. I searched everywhere in my New Testament for some mention of the Comforter. I found the dove— "And when Jesus was baptized, he went up immediately from the water, and behold, the heavens were opened and he saw the Spirit of God descending like a dove." *(Matthew 4:16)*—but no Comforter. I asked my minister about it, and she turned right to the page in John 14 where she knew this to be. No Comforter. Only Counselor. I was beginning to feel that I was searching for the elusive Holy Grail.

Aha. This is the Revised Standard Version. Perhaps the problem is one of translation. Reading the King James, I finally found the Comforter.

> *And I will pray the Father,*
> *and he shall give you another Comforter, that he may abide*
> *with you forever; . . .*
> *the Comforter, which is the Holy Ghost,*
> *whom the Father will send in my name, . . .*
> *shall teach you all things,*

and bring all things to your remembrance,
whatsoever I have said unto you.
Peace I leave with you, my peace I give unto you: . . .
Let not your heart be troubled, neither let it be afraid.

JOHN 14:16, 26–27

I tell the whole story because the change in translation from "Comforter" to "Counselor" seems so significant to me. When the word is read as "Counselor," the two parts of this passage seem separate. The first is about the Counselor, who will teach. The other is about God's peace. Two quite separate ideas. But read it as "Comforter," and the two parts flow together. The Comforter is the peace that Christ gives. The Comforter calms our fears and our troubled hearts. This is Christ's assurance, that in the midst of desolation, we will be comforted.

When we are in the midst of horror and despair, the last thing we want is to be counseled, that is, to be given advice. Though we do go to counselors—therapists, school guidance counselors, counselors-at-law—to guide us through times of distress, what we need at our times of deepest horror is comfort, mother love, to be held in empathic arms.

When my son, Paul, has been hurt, physically or emotionally, because of bad judgment on his part, I have been tempted, as I hold him, to make a lesson of this—to point out his mistakes, have him think how this happened to him and how he might avoid it in the future, but that is not what he wants or needs right then. Right then, he simply wants and needs to be held, to be told he's loved. The counseling can come later.

In my own moments of fear and horror, I crave comfort, touch. When advice is offered instead, I push it away, shut down, go farther into the pain. Comfort—being held, touched, listened to, sung to, tended with love and care—opens me up, helps me let go of the fear. Comforting is a way of giving and receiving the spirit. This maternal presence of the spirit/goddess reaches out to us in moments of despair and horror. Sometimes it comes through the touch of another. In the days, and especially the nights, before the transplant, I knew

153

such horror. How many times would I lie in the dark, listening to my heart beating erratically, wondering when I was going to explode, my fears chasing each other round and round, only to have them released into David's comforting arms around me. Or the times I would slip into tachycardia, and when I most needed to calm down, find myself gripped with anxiety, and then feel the reassurance of David's hand holding mine, bringing a spirit of calm to my heart and soul. One of my greatest moments of horror was the last long bout of shocking. The image still held vividly in my memory is of being jolted with the pain of the shocks, and of Nancy holding my hand, reassuring me with her touch and her words. Horror and comfort. I think it was Nancy's comforting presence that enabled me to relax just enough finally to convert my heart rhythm. Many extended hands of comfort to me—in the ambulance, in the recovery room, in CCU. (Doctors, I've noticed, want desperately to extend comfort, but also need to keep a doctor/patient boundary, so they tend to touch feet, hold toes, and yes, even that is comforting.) Even now as I go through biopsies, I often ask for a hand to hold, the comfort making the horror (which I reenter at every biopsy) endurable.

Though I held him more than he held me, my holding Paul was another source of comfort. There is a comfort in giving comfort, in holding close to the heart. It reminds me of the symbol for infinity. In my distress, or in his, the energy would loop around and out, seeking response. In our holding, in being held or in holding, the energy loops connect, forming a circuit, a mutual giving and receiving, a whole, an energy flow complete unto itself. In that holding, time does feel infinite, and yet not to exist at all. Holding, being held, a circle of comfort.

> *I want to hold the baby . . .*
> *I want to hold a baby.*
> *Let me hold the baby,*
> *even when it cries: cries*
> *and is still held,*
> *and cries and is held*
> *without rocking or*

pleading, cries
and is held,
is held, is held—
I want to be the large
and patient one,
and I want to be the one
with the tear-streaked face
within the cradle of arms.

MARISHA CHAMBERLAIN, "Let Me Hold the Baby"

I have known the dry, arid, harsh places of no comfort, no touch—times when I had gone so long without comfort that a single touch or a kind word would dissolve me into tears. They are hell indeed. Without comfort, without touch, something in us shrivels up and dies. Babies who are not touched die of malnutrition of the spirit. When I was first born and placed in an incubator, touched only to have my diaper changed, my spirit gave up and I refused to eat for four days. On the fourth day, a nurse broke regulations, took me out of the incubator, held me, rocked me, and in the comfort of those arms, life tasted sweet and I drank it in. Heaven is the place of mother love.

I often think one of the greatest horrors of leprosy, and its modern day equivalent—AIDS, is the refusal of touch. Certainly a person must shrivel up and die of that denial of the spirit sooner than of the disease itself. Christ, in touching the leper, extended to him the spirit of mother love, the spirit of the Comforter, so essential to our healing.

We can extend the spirit in so many ways. Our touch—comforting, healing touch—is one. But we also extend it through our words. So often, someone has spoken just the right words to me at just the right time, enabling me to get through times of horror, despair, disappointment. One of the transplant nurses, Sofia (also the name of the goddess of wisdom), comes particularly to mind as someone whose words of wisdom and consolation have often carried me over places of desolation. On my "dry run," Sofia was the one to tell me that the donor heart was not good enough. "We want you to be able to go to Paul's college graduation," she said. Just the right words to comfort me. She had created hope from disappointment. Again, on that horrible day in June when I was told I was rejecting, Sofia appeared just as I was entering the hospital corridor, and as I saw her the tears welled up in my eyes. "This is a little setback," she said. "I saw the biopsy report. It is a very minor rejection. We can fix it. Don't worry." And again, months later, when blood tests indicated a possible problem with my liver, and doctors hinted at the possibility of cancer, she took my hands and told me that she respected my fears, but now, "I want you to go envision yourself encircled with white light." And I did, and I was comforted. Words of comfort.

We can extend comfort through our listening. So many listened—my family, my friends. The transplant nurses are particularly skilled at listening—to pretransplant fears of whether the heart will come in time and to posttransplant fears of rejection, infection, cancer. They held, and continue to hold, me through it all with their willingness to listen.

We can extend comfort through music—

Music, oh sweet melody,
Won't you draw her close to you,
and comfort her for me.

MARGIE ADAM, "Having Been Touched" ("Tender Lady")

—that music sustained me throughout my ordeal; or we can extend comfort through our quiet, with simply a peaceful presence; and quite literally through our chicken soup. When people have fed me, made me food, in times of illness or despair, I have felt as fed by the comfort as by the food itself. It is the extension of the loving spirit that feeds us. We have so many ways to extend the spirit.

I have known horror throughout my ordeal, and I have been comforted through touch, song, nourishment of my body and soul.

Sometimes the maternal presence has come more directly as spirit. I think of the time I woke up in University Hospital, feeling held by hundreds of arms bathed in soothing white light. Even more did I feel this presence at those times of letting go into the moment of death, when I felt so held in such deep peace. "Peace I leave with you; my peace I give to you." Were the arms that held me the arms of the mother spirit, holding me one last time, easing my passage?

When I was twelve, I had a chance to see Michelangelo's *Pieta*. Never in all of my life have I been so deeply moved by a work of art. It touched something in my deepest core. What it was I didn't even try to figure out, but it strikes me now that that image of Mary, the mother holding the Christ child—but this time not as a babe, but as a dying man—evokes that mother spirit in the full circle of our lives. There was something so paradoxical, and so true, about that image of mother and child, so often associated with birth, now being associated with death. Life can hold such horrors, perhaps none so great as the moment of birth—of passage from the comfort of the womb into the cold dry bright loud world outside; and the moment of death—of passage from the comfort of the familiar into the harshness of the unknown (or at least we find horror in our fear of that passage, though perhaps it is simply a return to the mother—heaven as the womb.) In our death, as in our birth, we seek the comfort of being held in the arms of mother love. So also, in the little births and deaths—the risks, the changes, the various passages of our lives, we seek, and hopefully we find, comfort.

In the moment of reliving the greatest of my horrors, I had known comfort. Remembering that passage into death, I felt folded in the arms of my mother. "I will fold you in my arms like a white winged dove," sings Cris Williamson. In the passages of our lives, be they physical or spiritual, the dove, the spirit, the mother hears the cries of our spirit and folds us in her arms.

Born again

This, then, is salvation, when we marvel at the beauty of created things and praise the beautiful providence of their Creator.

MEISTER ECKHART

About eight months after my transplant, I was sitting at my kitchen table, looking out over Lake Superior, marveling at the beauty and splendor of it all, when I read this passage from one of Meister Eckhart's sermons. It was one of those "Aha!" moments, when suddenly something quite puzzling makes sense.

What had been puzzling to me was the notion of what it meant to be "born again." Throughout my life, various people near and dear to me have had this experience of being "born again." They had felt a grace, sometimes a chosenness by God, and had from that time devoted their lives to Christ. They believed in Christ as their salvation.

Maybe I hadn't experienced the grace, but I also never quite understood what it was we needed salvation from. I remember as a child, sitting in church, reading the prayer of confession, thinking, "I'm not this bad, horrible person this prayer says I am." I just couldn't quite get the idea of original sin.

Later, while a counselor at a mainstream Protestant church camp, I was faced with yet another encounter with this puzzling concept. It was a major turning point in my life. The camp that week had been filled with what were then termed "Jesus freaks"—people who had "found Christ" and were deeply into proselytizing. They had planned the communion service that week, and unlike any communion service of which I had ever been a part, we were each asked, upon receiving the bread and juice, whether we accepted Christ as our savior. Now, Christ and Christ's teachings were deeply in my heart, but I still didn't understand the savior part, so I could not honestly answer "yes" to that question. I turned and left without receiving communion. For a long time after that, I felt myself somewhat "excommunicated." I didn't believe in original sin; I didn't know what I thought about eternal life; I didn't believe Christ was the only way; I didn't want to believe in a Christianity that excluded other spiritual traditions; and I still didn't understand the whole idea of salvation.

Until now. This one passage from Eckhart made all of it make sense. This is salvation. This incredible marveling at the beauty of created things. Wonder.

And this wonder was available to me now in way that it never had been before because I was, quite literally, born again. Aha.

So this is what it means to be born again. To experience the world with the wonder that one has as a newborn babe. And I did. The colors seemed brighter. The air clearer. The sounds sweeter.

My six-year-old son tells me that everything is a miracle, and now, reborn, I can see that it is more clearly than I ever could before. A miracle that we can see the light of the stars billions of light years away—even the ones long dead; a miracle that we can eat a banana grown on a tree thousands of miles away; a miracle that by running our hands up and down piano keys, we can make of sound a melody that stirs the soul; a miracle that we can be warm even when the outside temperature is minus thirty degrees; a miracle that we can with the slightest variation in our facial muscles convey fear, anger, delight, disgust, sorrow, joy; a miracle that inside this tiny cell lies all of the information to grow a complete human being; a miracle that we can cut our finger and the skin grows back; a miracle that we can be so very angry and still love . . . it is all a miracle.

The two-year-old lives in a world of wonder. How many times did we turn the light on and off for my then two-year-old nephew, and each time watch him marvel and exclaim, "Light!" To take a walk with a two-year-old is to experience wonder. You don't get very far because everything becomes a possibility for discovery—the ants and the inchworm, the way a leaf has two different colors, the sparkling of bits of quartz crystals in a piece of granite, the squishiness of the mud, the way dirt balls explode on impact, the smells of the wild roses. And I think of my son, Paul, marveling at his own creation, looking in the mirror for hours, making faces, watching his body move, patting his tummy and saying "I you" (meaning "I love you") to his reflection.

> *A child's world is fresh and new and beautiful, full of*
> *wonder and excitement. It is our misfortune that for most*
> *of us that clear-eyed vision, that true instinct for what is*
> *beautiful and awe-inspiring, is dimmed and even lost*
> *before we reach adulthood. If I had influence with the*
> *good fairy who is supposed to preside over the christening*
> *of all children I should ask that her gift to each child in the*
> *world be a sense of wonder so indestructible that it would*
> *last throughout life, as an unfailing antidote against the*
> *boredom and disenchantments of later years,*
> *the sterile preoccupation with things that are artificial,*
> *the alienation from the sources of our strength.*
>
> RACHEL CARSON, *The Sense of Wonder*

Perhaps this more than anything was the exquisite gift of this new heart—the gift of an indestructible sense of wonder. It literally allowed me to be born again—to experience the world as I did when I was first born, but with the awareness and the capacity for reflection and communication that I did not have as a child. Now, born again to this two-year-old sense of wonder, I too could marvel at the beauty of all of creation. In those first few months after the transplant, I found it hard to sleep, so enthralled was I with the beauty of it all. I didn't want to miss a moment. Not a sunrise, not a sunset, not a moonrise, not a thunderstorm, not a hawk passing overhead, not the changing colors of the lake, not a single star—and the marvels of "nature" were just the beginning. I marveled at the way I could move my body again and at the way it could feel physically tired at the end of the day. I marveled at all the ideas that were bursting forth in me. I felt so creative—so many projects, ideas, thoughts all coming together. There were so many marvelous books to read—what a wonder that there were so many ideas in the world. I kept myself awake with the marvel of all the life that lay ahead of me—all the hills to climb, the garden to grow, the lake that begged to be swum in. I needed hours just to contemplate the clouds. All of it seemed so much more beautiful and marvelous and miraculous than I had ever known.

With the wonder came also the praise of which Eckhart speaks, for how could I experience this wonder and not feel blessed, and for this blessing I was so deeply grateful and humbled. And I celebrated. So much of what I had learned—the mindfulness, gratitude, humility, joy, celebration—came together in this experience of wonder and praise. Surely this was salvation.

As deeply as I marveled at the beauty of creation, so much more profoundly have I been affected by our neglect and squandering of it, by our capacity and inclination to destroy all of this. I have felt more deeply the sting of the destructive capacities of greed, ambition, envy, hatred. If there is an original sin, it seems it must be this—a separation from our sense of wonder, from the genuine childlike appreciation of the marvel of all of creation—a separation that allows us to squander, neglect, and destroy these great gifts, in ourselves and in the world. If there is a salvation, of ourselves, of our species, it seems it must begin here, with an immersion in the marvel and wonder. No one who truly appreciated the marvel of their mind and body could willingly destroy it with drugs or mindless video games or pesticide-ridden food. No one who truly appreciated the marvel of the clear waters could dump toxic chemicals in them. No one who truly appreciated the marvel of the soil could burn it out with fertilizer or simply let it erode away. No one who truly appreciated the marvel of their own special genius would willingly let it be destroyed in mind-numbing work or destructive relationships.

Living in wonder brings forth reverence, for all created things. All are held sacred. In this wonder and this reverencing of all of creation lies the beginning of salvation.

We are one

Nothing is precious
except that part of you which is in other people
and that part of others which is in you.
Up there
on high,
everything is one.

PIERRE TEILHARD DE CHARDIN

Before the transplant, people would often ask me how I felt about having another person's heart inside my body. Of all the things surrounding the transplant—the operation, cutting my heart out, the possibility of rejection and infection, even the waiting for someone to die that I might live—this, having someone else's heart inside my body, was the thing that seemed most disturbing to people. As it was to me.

What would it be like to have a part of another person inside of me? Didn't that violate something? Don't we have skin around us, separating each from the other, for a reason? But more than this, I wondered whether I would be different somehow after the transplant. I wondered whether I would indeed lose a part of myself and become, in part, another person.

We were talking about my heart, the part of my body most central to my identity. How could I lose my heart and not be different?

165

Language, culture, and spiritual traditions taught that my heart was the core of my loving. With my heart gone, with someone else's heart, would I love in the same way? Would I love the same people? Though on some level I thought my questions to be foolish, on another I feared I would no longer love my husband, or even my child, with another's heart in me.

Would my questions and fears have been different if it were my kidney or liver that was to be replaced? I don't identify myself so deeply with those organs. Yet others I have known with transplanted kidneys and livers have had similar questions.

All in all, I feared for the integrity of my being.

Several things helped in my coming to terms with this. The most immediate was my experience of pregnancy. I had known what it was to have another person, and not just a part, a whole person, growing inside my body. It did not feel foreign to me. I did not feel invaded. This other life inside me was a joy. We were in this life together. Indeed, it was the separation rather than the joining that was difficult.

As I prepared for the transplant, I reminded myself of this experience, and after the transplant, I held this new heart in my mind's eye as if in my womb. I wanted to welcome it, to nurture and protect it, as if it were my child. And it seemed medically prudent, since pregnancy is the one time that the body will accept a foreign body, even one with a different blood type, without attacking it with T-cells and white cells. It was important that we become one.

Yet even in pregnancy, the two, though connected, are separate. Each has its own identity. How to be connected and yet my own person? In the process of my attempts at self-healing, I became aware of the several layers of self/body/mind, the physical body being only one—the etheric, astral, and spiritual bodies being separate yet interconnected systems. So even if I had another's physical heart, my astral heart and spiritual heart energies were still my own—or at least so I reasoned. My understanding was limited, but enough to make some sense of what would change in me and what would not.

The main insight that brought peace to my questioning was a friend's statement: "You know, Beth, we are all one." I'm not sure exactly what that meant to me at the time. I just know that it spoke to a basic truth in me, and that it resonated with the scientific theories and the spiritual traditions that touched my heart.

As a young child, my brother, the budding physicist, would amaze me with his statements. "All the atoms in the world are the same ones that were here thousands, millions of years ago. You may be breathing the same particles of air that Plato breathed. In fact, if we put all the atoms together right, we could hear his words." I was made of the same atoms as people living thousands of years ago. So were the trees and the grass and the lakes. We're all made of the same stuff. I was wonderstruck.

> "We are all made of the same stuff, remember, we of the Jungle, you of the City. The same substance composes us—the tree overhead,
> the stone beneath us, the bird, the beast, the star—
> we are all one, all moving to the same end.
> Remember that when you no longer remember me, my child."
>
> "But how can tree be stone? A bird is not me.
> Jane is not a tiger," said Michael stoutly.
>
> "You think not?" said the Hamadryad's hissing voice.
> "Look!" and he nodded his head towards the moving mass of creatures before them. Birds and animals were now swaying together, closely encircling Mary Poppins, who was rocking lightly from side to side. Backwards and forwards went the swaying crowd, keeping time together, swinging like the pendulum of a clock. Even the trees were bending and lifting gently, and the moon seemed to be rocking in the sky as a ship rocks on the sea.
>
> "Bird and beast and stone and star—we are all one, all one—
> . . ."

P. L. TRAVERS, *Mary Poppins*

Later in my life, popular accounts of physics also left me in amazement. Over and over again, scientific theories bore out this same truth that we are one. According to David Bohm's notion of implicate order, all of reality is contained within each of its parts. Bell's theorem mathematically "proves" that subatomic particles are connected in such a way that whatever happens to one particle immediately affects the others. Rupert Sheldrake's hypothesis of morphogenesis extends Bell's theorem to changes in species behavior. In the true story of "the hundredth monkey," after the hundredth monkey on an isolated island in the Pacific had learned to wash the sand off potatoes before eating them, monkeys on other islands spontaneously began washing their potatoes as well. The distinctions between us blur.

> *Most amazing is this realization that everything that exists in the universe came from a common origin. The material of your body and the material of my body are intrinsically related because they emerged from and are caught up in a single energetic event.*
>
> *Our ancestry stretches back through the life forms and into the stars, back to the beginnings of the primeval fireball. This universe is a single multiform energetic unfolding of matter, mind, intelligence, and life.*
>
> BRIAN SWIMME, *The Universe Is a Green Dragon*

I found similar conclusions in a variety of philosophical and spiritual traditions as well. Buddhism, Hinduism, Taoism, Christianity, Transcendentalism, Romanticism, medieval mysticism, Native American traditions—all speak of the interconnectedness of all beings, of being one in the spirit.

I didn't totally rationally comprehend all the scientific or mystical explanations, but I knew in my heart that my friend's wisdom was true. The distinctions we make between our bodily selves, drawn by the boundaries of our bodies/psyches, do seem somewhat arbitrary. We are both separate and distinct and never wholly so. We all came from the same source. Our souls resonate with the same energies. In our unions we find reunion. The union of this heart with my body would simply be that—a reunion, a reminder of the interconnectedness of all life.

After the transplant, people were very curious. They'd heard the same stories I had, of people developing strange cravings for food or longings for particular kinds of music. Had I experienced that? What was it like to have another person's heart beating in my body? Did I feel different? Could I sense her presence? Was I like J. now?

I first began wondering about the effects of this new connection as I awoke from my anesthesia stupor, only to be plagued with horror-filled hallucinations and nightmares. On an intellectual level, I knew the nightmares and hallucinations were probably drug-induced, but they were so intense and so horrific that, on a deeper level, I felt I was experiencing the cries of a soul in torment. I wondered what kind of horror this child, whose heart now beat in me, had known—perhaps in her dying. I wondered if she were rebelling at being placed in a strange body. All my fears had been of my rejecting her; perhaps she was rejecting me.

A few days later, as I began to more fully recover my faculties, I could actually feel the heart beating inside me. That is a major difference between a transplanted heart and a transplanted liver or kidney or pancreas, whose presence is not so obvious and felt. This heart I could feel, beating, alive within me. It was much smaller than my old heart, and placed slightly higher in my body, so it felt somewhat out of place. And it was very fast. This new heart was twice as fast as my old one, beating at a speed that in my previous life would have set off my defibrillator. This rapid pace was shocking in its own way.

Yet I was surprised how quickly I settled into the new rhythm. The heart was fast, but steady. Never in my adult life had I known such a steady beat. It felt good, and I felt confident.

My new heart is steady, smooth. I have almost come to take it for granted. Such a luxury—this freedom from fear. Such a gift.

MARCH 15, 1994

I felt very protective of my new heart, especially on that day shortly after my transplant when they invaded it for the biopsy.

———⦿———

On Thursday they took four snips of the inside of it. I felt as if I were holding it all during the biopsy—telling it we'd get through this together.

MARCH 6, 1994

I didn't want anyone messing with my new heart. It seemed so young and vulnerable and so perfect to me, and it had been placed in my care. I still feel that way. I want to do all that I can to keep it healthy, to carry us both through this life.

The word that best described my feeling towards this new heart—far from estranged or invaded—was sympatico. I felt our two hearts (I do indeed still have a sense of my old heart within me.) beating as one, and felt that our souls touched and met in reunion. Indeed, the most astonishing thing to me, on a spiritual level, about my episode of rejection was that it could have happened at all.

———⦿———

I do love this heart. Why am I rejecting it? I frankly thought that was an impossibility. I feel so sympatico with this heart.

JUNE 11, 1994

I felt sympatico, but not particularly changed. To the disappointment of the curious, I have not developed new tastes. My essential personality, sometimes to my regret, is basically the same as it was before the transplant. I am glad to say that I still love my husband and son and family and friends as before. I do, from time to time, have a sense of J.'s presence with me. As I have written, I sometimes felt that it was J.'s grief rather than my own that gripped my soul. And it is healing to me to know that J. was so beloved and so loving, such a joy to all who knew her. Somehow I hope that some of that will rub off on me. But basically I feel myself the same as before the transplant.

And yet not. I feel that I am walking this life with someone in a way I did not previously. My doctor once asked me how I felt about my new heart. Did it feel like my heart? Like J.'s heart? I told him neither. I felt that we shared it. I still do. This feels like a collaborative venture. As the old song goes:

From thee I receive
To thee I give
Together we share
That both may live.

Immediately after the transplant, I knew little of my donor, only that it was a nine-year-old child. After some time, I began a correspondence with my donor's family and slowly learned more of J. and her life. As I have come to know more about J., I have felt both more removed from her and more connected—seeing her as a separate person with a life separate and apart from mine, and yet knowing her more intimately by knowing something of her.

I look at the pictures of J. I read the letters from her parents and her aunt. I see and feel and taste and touch the interweavings of lives and know that we all help each other to go on. J. will always be in my heart. She is indeed precious to me. What exactly we know of each other, me of her, she of me, the ways we change and grow together, seem both so clear and yet so mysterious. My husband, wondering about all these things, expressed the essence of it in a song:

did she walk down by the sea
was the sorrow in her way
were her hands held toward the breeze
did she feel the sun that rose to warm her hair
to stir the blood that ran her veins
yesterday she cast a shadow
now today we share her name
will your eyes look on this harbor
will your ears be filled with mine
if I stand a little closer

will you be there
will you pass your secrets to me
with the wind that whispers by
with the sun that dances over
and with the line above which it rises
when my hand grips on the hoe
as my feet step on this path
I'll remember what I'm growing
I'll always know the places I have found you sleeping
deep in dreams that do not last
the destiny that holds our wishes
and the names that issue from the past
all at once we'll follow over
all of us and all the same
but still we stop to tell the stories
of all the love and all the service
all the joys and all the pain
all the plans and all the failures
of every warm inviting rain
that falls in shadows cast on roses
mourned by any other name

DAVE WINCHESTER

The questions posed by a transplant, by placing the very heart of one into the body of another, are age-old. What is the seat of our personality? Of our memory? Of our tastes and talents and desires? Of our soul? Are they contained in our bodies? In particular parts of our bodies? If I take on a part of another body, do I take on that person as well? What is the intertwining of body/mind/soul? I don't know that I have discovered any particular answers. It is still a great mystery.

I do know that my thoughts and fears of a violation of the integrity of my self seem folly now, incidental to the larger scheme of things. The interconnectedness of it all, of all our lives, is what I live.

Open heart

Whenever your heart is broken, you receive a blessing—
your broken heart becomes an open heart.

DOUGLAS BLOCH

———— ❧ ————

"You're rejecting," they say. And I want to respond, "No, I'm protecting." My body is responding just as it should, protecting me from what it regards as a hostile and dangerous invader. But it has misperceived. This heart needs protection, too. So I draw a circle of protection around it with my mind. Keep it safe.

Rejection. It's a horrible word. Full of disapproval, failure, relationships gone bad, publishers' refusals, nonacceptance, refusal to admit, to permit, to allow entry, to give a chance—a refusal of love.

To die of rejection. The shriveling of the heart. No one deserves such a fate. Yet how many shrivel up a little every day— at the little rejections, the slights, the conditions we put on our love. The little deaths of the spirit.

To learn to love unconditionally. That is our task. Is it the lesson I need to learn here? I have been so critical lately. Every *criticism entails a rejection—not good enough—foolish—stu-pid—wrong.*

The pain of rejection. Devastation. A wasteland. Gasping for breath. Weakness. Fatigue. Erosion of the soul.

It demands reclamation. Don't let them do that to you. Don't let them tell you your work your life your looks your love aren't good enough. Love your heart, your body, your mind, your spirit. Love with the heart wide open.

Believe. Trust. Affirm. The universe is benevolent.

JUNE 11, 1994

Four months after my transplant, one week after my heartwarming celebration to welcome this new heart, a few hours after I had told David, "I'm so happy, I hardly know what to do," Mary from the transplant center called to tell me I was rejecting. Rejecting. That meant my immune system was attacking my heart, trying to kill off the invader—doing its job, yes, but my perfectly functioning immune system was killing me. It is a tricky balance—immunosuppression. Too much and my body sickens with infection; too little and I risk rejection. The trick is to stay open to the healing powers and yet remain protected from rejection.

I returned to the hospital, where they pumped my body with one thousand milligrams of IV prednisone, which would keep my army of white cells at bay. They stopped the rejection, but now that vague possibility of rejection was a reality, and I lost my trust.

So here I am wondering again how much time I have left. Are these my last few weeks of life? It is so bizarre when I feel so fine, yet I know that if this doesn't reverse, I'll die soon. . . .

They say this is just a temporary setback. I have to believe them. I want years and years.

And yet the bizarre twist is that the world seems poised on the brink of nuclear war tonight. Will any of us last out the week? . . . I fear for us all.

I don't ever want to take life for granted, but I want to take living for granted. I want to be able to assume a future. I want to be able to live without the omnipresent weight of my mortality.

It was so nice, those few weeks, to scan my life for that feeling that something is really wrong—and find it gone. For a short while all was right with the world. Even if I survive this episode, will I ever regain trust in that again?

How to trust in a benevolent universe?

JUNE 14, 1994

Before this, rejection had been a theoretical possibility, but one I had not taken very seriously. Now it was real, and the reality of rejection was devastating and eye opening. Despite the miracle of this new heart and this new life, I could still die at any time. I wasn't safe. I wasn't cured. I wasn't immortal. I had just graciously been given some more time, and that gift could be taken away from me at any time.

Part of me wanted to close off, protect every inch of the precious space in front of me. Close out the world, the demands, the stresses, the pain and suffering. Claim this safe place as mine, a protected shell. But this was where my heart journey had started—closed off, walled away, damming up my heart—fearing its rejection. Had I come all this way just to come full circle?

No. This was not the lesson I had to learn—rather, I needed to open, to embrace with an open heart. Trust, affirm, flow, let go, live in gratitude and joy and celebration.

Fear of rejection had closed me off the first time.

Fear of rejection nearly had kept me from opting for this new heart and all of its blessings.

Fear of rejection was simply that—fear. It would not change the possibility of rejection. There was no way to protect myself. The possibility of rejection will be with me, ever present, the rest of my life. Always will there be a reminder of the tenuousness and the preciousness of life.

The lesson of rejection is not to close. No amount of closing out the world will protect me from rejection. No, the lesson of rejection, paradoxically, is to open. To live well with the time remaining. To live and love with an open heart.

What is it to love with an open heart? Not to reject—any thought, any person, any aspect of myself. Unconditional acceptance. Forgiveness. Trust. Radical empathy. Compassion.

It requires what Sam Keen calls metanoia—the opposite of paranoia—to turn around and "reown the shadow"—to recognize that all of the qualities of humanity, the good and the bad, the dark and the light—love, compassion, kindness, hatred, evil, envy, fear, violence—are in ourselves as much as in anyone.

> . . . *To be twice-born,* [interesting that he would use that phrase]
> *I must face my own hostility, my fear, my rage, my disappointment,*
> *my resentment, my anxiety, my boredom, my terror,*
> *my helplessness, my confusion, my ambivalence.*
> *All of the rejected images flood into my consciousness. . . .*
> *When I know my shadow, I know that "they" are like me.*
> *We share a common human nature. The 50 percent of the human race*
> *I cast into the category of aliens are fellow humans who, like myself,*
> *are faulted, filled with contradictory impulses of love and hate,*
> *generosity, and a blind will to survive. . . . Metanoia brings the enemy within the circle of co-promising, conversation, and compassion.*
>
> SAM KEEN, *The Passionate Life*

Rejections. My rejections—of violence, bigotry, waste, impatience, ingratitude, miserliness—are real, and I struggle with them. I can appall myself with my harshness and my judgmentalism—my rejections. And then does my judgment turn back upon myself, so continuing the pattern, for most likely my harshness towards others stems from my harshness towards myself. Love your enemy . . . and your neighbor as yourself. Are they not one and the same? The things I hate in "the enemy" are most often those things I hate in myself, so that in learning to love and accept them in myself, I can learn to love and accept them in my enemy. That does not mean that I have to condone violence and bigotry, but that I recognize their source well enough that I can treat them mercifully, with compassion. If I am more loving, more patient, more kind, less resentful, less violent than another, it is not that I am better, just more fortunate. I could be and am all of these. As Thich Nhat Hanh says so well:

I am the mayfly metamorphosing on the surface of the river.
and I am the bird, which, when spring comes,
arrives in time to eat the mayfly.
I am a frog swimming happily in the clear water of a pond,
and I am also the grass-snake who,
approaching in silence, feeds itself on the frog.
I am the child in Uganda, all skin and bones,
my legs as thin as bamboo sticks.
and I am the arms merchant,
selling deadly weapons to Uganda.
I am the twelve-year-old girl, refugee
on a small boat,
who throws herself into the ocean after
being raped by a sea pirate,
and I am the pirate, my heart not yet capable
of seeing and loving.
I am a member of the politburo, with
plenty of power in my hands,
and I am the man who has to pay his
"debt of blood" to my people,
dying slowly in a forced labor camp.
My joy is like spring, so warm it makes
flowers bloom in all walks of life.
My pain is like a river of tears, so full it
fills up the four oceans.

Please call me by my true names,
so I can hear all my cries
and my laughs at once,
so I can see that my joy and pain are one.
Please call me by my true names,
so I can wake up,
and so the door of my heart can be left open,
the door of compassion.

THICH NHAT HANH, "Please Call Me by My True Names"

Compassion—leaving the door to the heart open.

Open, and yet protected, that is the balance, for the flip side of rejection is infection, disease. And what of my impulse to close, to claim these days as sacred, inviolable—when I have already missed so much, when I owe so much, when there is only so much time? It too needs to be honored as it comes. I need to accept my need to close off now and then, close down, draw a circle of protection around my heart, rest. Rest is good for the heart. I don't expect I would want to stay closed forever. To stay open and protected—that's the trick, the paradox in which I live.

———— ∾ ————

My sense is that I will be fine. I need to live. I want to live,
and live well.

JUNE 11, 1994

What is this impulse, this vision, this sense of purpose, vitality, destiny that fills me with this great desire to live?

The words that keep coming to my mind are these:

YOUTH: What is our fullest destiny?
THOMAS: To become love in human form.

BRIAN SWIMME, *The Universe Is a Green Dragon*

Yes, this rings true. Actually, it was a lesson I learned long ago as I faced my mortality in my early twenties. It being quite clear to me at the time that life was short and could be snatched away from me at any time, I pondered often what life was all about, that it could end so quickly. The only thing that made sense to me was love. Loving relationships. To become love in human form.

It seems so simple, almost trite. I even found the message on my box of Celestial Seasonings tea this morning:

> *Love is what we were born with. Fear is what we learn.*
> *The spiritual journey is the unlearning of fear and the*
> *acceptance of love back into our hearts. Love is the essential*
> *reality and our purpose on earth. To be consciously aware of*
> *it, to experience love in ourselves, is the meaning of life.*
>
> MARIANNE WILLIAMSON, *A Return to Love*
> (Celestial Seasonings—Orange Mango Zinger)

And yet it is not simple. To become love. How do we do that? The lesson of rejection is to open the heart. And how do we open the heart? I have only fragments of wisdom. This book has been about openings. Mindfulness, gratitude, letting go, hope, humility, forgiveness, joy, wonder—each is a path, a path to open the heart.

> *Love your heart, your body, your mind, your spirit.*
> *Love with the heart wide open.*
> *Believe. Trust. Affirm. The universe is benevolent.*

Credits

Page 30   From *Siddhartha* by Herman Hesse. Copyright © 1951 by New Directions Pub. Corp. Reprinted by permission of New Directions.

Page 35   Excerpted, with permission, from *The Creation of Health* by Caroline Myss and Dr. Norman Shealy. The book was published in 1988 by Stillpoint Publishing International, Inc. in Walpole, NH and is available by calling 1-800-847-4014.

Page 40   From *Healing Into Life and Death* by Stephen Levine. Reprinted with permission of Doubleday, a division of Bantam Doubleday Dell Publishing Group, Inc.

Page 56   Reprinted from *Sister Outsider* by Audre Lorde. Copyright © 1984, with permission of The Crossing Press, Freedom, California.

Page 73   From *Women Who Run with the Wolves: Myths and Stories of the Wild Woman Archetype* by Clarissa Pinkola Estes. Reprinted with permission of Ballantine Books, a Division of Random House Inc.

Page 75   From *The Miracle of Mindfulness* by Thich Nhat Hanh. Reprinted with permission of Beacon Press.

Page 76   From *The Miracle of Mindfulness* by Thich Nhat Hanh. Reprinted with permission of Beacon Press.

Page 79   Reprinted from *Being Peace* by Thich Nhat Hanh (1987) with permission of Parallax Press, Berkeley, California.

Page 82   "Replenish," used by permission of Claudia Schmidt

Page 84   From *Anne Frank: The Diary of a Young Girl* by Anne Frank, translated by B. M. Mooyart. Reprinted with permission of Doubleday, a division of Bantam Doubleday Dell Publishing Group, Inc.

Page 85   From *Disturbing the Peace: A Conversation with Karel Hvizdala* by Vaclav Havel, Karel Hvizdala, translated by Paul Wilson. © 1990. Reprinted with permission of Alfred A Knopf Inc.

Page 86   From *Anne Frank: The Diary of a Young Girl* by Anne Frank, translated by B. M. Mooyart. Reprinted with permission of Doubleday, a division of Bantam Doubleday Dell Publishing Group, Inc.

Page 88   From *Anne Frank: The Diary of a Young Girl* by Anne Frank, translated by B. M. Mooyart. Reprinted with permission of Doubleday, a division of Bantam Doubleday Dell Publishing Group, Inc.

Page 89   "Replenish," used by permission of Claudia Schmidt

Page 91   From *Letters to a Young Poet* by Rainer Maria Rilke, translated by M. D. Herter Norton. Translation copyright 1934, 1954 by W. W. Norton & Company, Inc. renewed © 1962, 1982 by M. D. Herter Norton. Reprinted by permission of W. W. Norton & Company, Inc.

Page 99   From *Way of the Peaceful Warrior* by Dan Millman. Copyright © 1984, published by HJ Kramer Inc.

Page 101   From *Open Mind, Open Heart: The Contemplative Dimension of the Gospel* by Thomas Keating. Copyright © 1986, published by Amity House.

Page 121   Words and music by Cris Williamson, © 1975 Bird Ankles Music (BMI) used by permission.

Page 130   From *Lyrical and Critical Essays* by Albert Camus, translated by Ellen Kennedy, © 1970. Reprinted with permission of Alfred A Knopf Inc., New York.

Page 134   Words and music by Cris Williamson, © 1975 Bird Ankles Music (BMI) used by permission.

Page 137   From *Breakthrough: Meister Eckhart's Creation Spirituality in New Translation,* translated by Matthew Fox, © 1980. Reprinted with permission of Doubleday, a division of Bantam Doubleday Dell Publishing Group, Inc.

Page 143   Words and music by Cris Williamson, © 1975 Bird Ankles Music (BMI) used by permission.

Page 149   Words and music by Cris Williamson, © 1975 Bird Ankles Music (BMI) used by permission.

Page 154   From "Let Me Hold the Baby" by Marisha Chamberlain. Used by permission.

Page 156   "Tender Lady," used by permission of Margie Adam, Labyris Music Co. ASCAP.

Page 161   Quote from *The Sense of Wonder* by Rachel Carson. Photographs by Charles Pratt. Copyright © renewed 1984 by Roger Christie. Reprinted by permission of HarperCollins Publishers, Inc.

Page 167   Reprinted from *Mary Poppins* by P. L. Travers, published by Harcourt Brace and Company.

Page 168   From *The Universe Is a Green Dragon: A Cosmic Creation Story* by Brian Swimme. Copyright © 1985, published by Bear & Co.

Page 173   From *Words that Heal* by Douglas Bloch, © 1988. Reprinted with permission of Bantam Doubleday Dell Publishing Group, Inc.

Page 176   From *The Passionate Life: Stages of Loving* by Sam Keen, ©1983 by Sam Keen. Reprinted with permission of HarperCollins Publishers.

Page 177   "Please Call Me by My True Names." Reprinted from *Being Peace* by Thich Nhat Hanh (1987) with permission of Parallax Press, Berkeley, California.

Page 178   From *The Universe Is a Green Dragon: A Cosmic Creation Story* by Brian Swimme. Copyright © 1985, published by Bear & Co.

Page 179   Reprinted from *A Return to Love* by Marianne Williamson. Copyright © 1992 by Marianne Williamson with permission of HarperCollins Publishers, New York.

NOTE: All Bible selections (except those on pages 152 and 153, which are from the King James version) are from the *Revised Standard Version of the Bible,* copyright 1946 and 1952 by the Division of Christian Education of the National Council of the Churches of Christ in the USA. Used by permission. All rights reserved.

Pfeifer-Hamilton Publishers produces quality gift books
celebrating the special beauty and unique lifestyle of the north country.

Christine Clifford
Not Now . . . I'm Having a No Hair Day

Eve Shaw
Grandmother's Alphabet

Laura Erickson
Sharing the Wonder of Birds with Kids
For the Birds

Jeff Hagen
Steeple Chase

Bob Cary
Tales from Jackpine Bob
Root Beer Lady

Shirley Babior, LCSW, MFCC
Carol Goldman, LICSW
Overcoming Panic, Anxiety, & Phobias

Donald A. Tubesing, PhD
Nancy Loving Tubesing, EdD
Seeking Your Healthy Balance
Kicking Your Holiday Stress Habits

Donald A. Tubesing, PhD
Kicking Your Stress Habits

Leigh Anne Jasheway, MPH
Don't Get Mad, Get Funny!

Call us toll free at 800-247-6789 for a complete catalog.

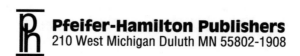

Pfeifer-Hamilton Publishers
210 West Michigan Duluth MN 55802-1908